Better than expected?!

Why persons with congenital heart disease can have a better quality of life than healthy people

Philip Moons

Copyright © 2011 by Heart vzw

All rights reserved. No part of this book may be reproduced, stored in a retrieval system, or transmitted in any form or by any means, electronic, mechanical, photocopying, recording, or otherwise, without prior permission of the author.

ISBN: 978-90-818248-0-4
NUR: 882

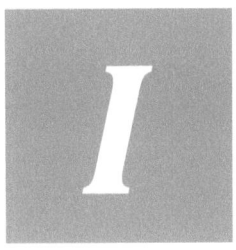

Contents

Contents	I
Permissions	II
Preface	III
Abbreviations	IV

Chapter 1   1
The quality of quality-of-life studies in congenital heart disease

Chapter 2   17
Quality of life: what is it and what is being measured?

Chapter 3   25
Quality of life of adults with congenital heart disease is better than that of healthy counterparts

Chapter 4   37
Individual quality of life of adults with congenital heart disease: What is important for their quality of life?

Chapter 5   53
Quality of life of adults with congenital heart disease is marginally associated with disease severity

Chapter 6   67
Profile of adults with congenital heart disease having a good, moderate, or poor quality of life

Chapter 7   79
Sense of coherence as a pathway to explain why patients with congenital heart disease have a better quality of life

Epilogue   87

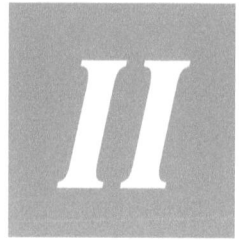

Permissions

Each of the following articles has been reprinted with permission of the publisher.

Chapter 1
Moons P, Van Deyk K, Budts W, De Geest S. Caliber of quality-of-life studies in congenital heart disease: A plea for more conceptual and methodological rigor. Archives of Pediatrics & Adolescent Medicine 2004; 158: 1062-1069. *(Copyright © (2004) American Medical Association. All rights reserved)*

Chapter 3
Moons P, Van Deyk K, De Bleser L, Marquet K, Raes E, De Geest S, Budts W. Quality of life and health status in adults with congenital heart disease: A direct comparison with healthy counterparts. European Journal of Cardiovascular Prevention and Rehabilitation 2006; 13: 407-413. *(Copyright © (2006) Sage Publications Ltd./Inc. All rights reserved)*

Chapter 4
Moons P, Van Deyk K, Marquet K, Raes E, De Bleser L, Budts W, De Geest S. Individual quality of life of adults with congenital heart disease: A paradigm shift. European Heart Journal 2005; 26: 298-307. *(Copyright © (2005) Oxford University Press. All rights reserved)*

Chapter 5
Moons P, Van Deyk K, De Geest S, Gewillig M, Budts W. Is severity of congenital heart disease associated with the quality of life and perceived health of adult patients? Heart, 2005; 91: 1193-1198. *(Copyright © (2005) BMJ Publishing Group, Ltd. All rights reserved)*

Chapter 6
Moons P, Van Deyk K, Marquet K, De Bleser L, De Geest S, Budts W. Profile of adults with congenital heart disease with a good, moderate or poor quality of life: A cluster analytic study. European Journal of Cardiovascular Nursing 2009, 8: 151-157. *(Copyright © (2009) Elsevier. All rights reserved)*

Chapter 7
Moons P, Norekvål TM. Is sense of coherence a pathway to improve the quality of life of patients who grow up with chronic diseases? A hypothesis. European Journal of Cardiovascular Nursing 2006; 5: 16-20. *(Copyright © (2009) Elsevier. All rights reserved)*

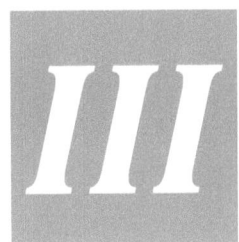

Preface

The number of persons with congenital heart disease in society is continuously growing, owing to an increased life expectancy. To date, about 90% of children born with congenital heart disease can reach adulthood. Due to the increased life expectancy, issues beyond the quantity of life have become relevant. In this respect, studies have been conducted on patient's illness perception, such as perceived health status, functional status and quality of life. Such studies have found that persons with congenital heart disease may have physical impediments. Based on these observations, researchers sometimes assume that individuals with congenital heart disease have a diminished quality of life. However, this does not fit with clinical impressions that a large portion of persons with congenital heart disease have a good quality of life. The paradox of having physical limitations, albeit experiencing an excellent quality of life urges us to raise some questions: How well are studies on quality of life in congenital heart disease methodologically conducted? How is quality of life defined and measured? Can patients indicate what they think is important for their quality of life? How can a good quality of life in persons with congenital heart disease be explained?

An extensive research program on quality of life in congenital heart disease has been established at the Center for Health Services and Nursing Research of the Katholieke Universiteit Leuven (Belgium) in collaboration with the Adult Congenital Heart Disease program of the University Hospitals Leuven (Belgium). This book describes the results of the different studies that have been conducted in this respect. Hence, this book is a source for clinicians and researchers to understand how persons with congenital heart disease can have an excellent quality of life, despite some physical impediments. It provides a scientific basis that can guide future studies. Furthermore, this book can be a source of support for patients and parents to value a good quality of life, irrespective the heart condition. Indeed, the quality of life of persons with congenital heart disease is influenced by many other things than the heart condition.

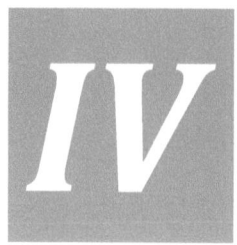

Abbreviations

AICD: Automatic Implantable Cardioverter Defibrillator
ASD: Atrial Septal Defect
CHD-TAAQOL: TNO-AZL Adult Quality of Life – Congenital Heart Disease
EQ-5D: Euroqol 5 dimensions
H: Hypothesis
ICC: Intra Class Correlation
IQR: Inter Quartile Range
LAS: Linear Analog Scale
NYHA: New York Heart Association
Q1: Quartile 1
Q3: Quartile 3
QoL: Quality of life
SEIQoL Schedule for the Evaluation of Quality of Life: SEIQoL-DW
Schedule for the Evaluation of Quality of Life – Direct Weighting
SF-36, 36 item short form health survey
SPSS: Statistical Package for Social Sciences
SWLS: Satisfaction with Life Scale
VSD: Ventricular Septal Defect

Chapter 1

The quality of quality-of-life studies in congenital heart disease

During the past decades, mortality in congenital heart disease has decreased significantly.[1,2] However, specific social and psychological concerns that typically occur in patients as they advance through life, such as compromised employability, insurability, and declining social integration,[3-5] have caused health care professionals and researchers to take notice of the effect of this change. To substantiate a differentiated view on the outcomes of this patient population, the quality of life in patients with congenital heart disease has increasingly been addressed. Information on quality of life allows us to gain a better understanding of relevant issues for these patients, which is essential for optimizing their clinical management, planning appropriate care, and evaluating specific interventions or therapeutic modes.

Although quality-of life research has grown exponentially, major conceptual and methodological challenges have also emerged. Indeed, consensus still eludes us regarding the conceptualization, operational definition, and measurement of quality of life. Because of this, quality of life is often incorrectly used as a generic label to describe a range of physical and psychosocial variables, making it an umbrella term that covers a variety of concepts, such as functioning, health status, perceptions, life conditions, behavior, happiness, lifestyle, symptoms, etc.[6] The lack of a uniform definition for quality of life contributes to its conceptual vagueness and obscurity.

Obviously, interpretation of results from quality-of-life studies becomes complicated when investigators do not use a consistent conceptual basis to define quality of life or if they fail to even define quality of life. This uneven, inappropriate usage, for instance, sometimes leads researchers to conclude that patients have a good quality of life just because they are employed,[7] do not report symptoms or require medication,[8] or are not in need of reoperation.[9] This problem was recognized by Gill and Feinstein[10] in their landmark study that assessed the caliber of quality-of-life measurements in different populations of patients. Using 10 criteria (see "Review Criteria and Procedure" subsection of the "Methods" section) specifically developed for use in their evaluation of 75 randomly selected quality-of-life studies, they concluded that most quality-of-life measurements and studies required methodological improvement because they "aimed at the wrong target."[10(p619)]

The purpose of this article is to critically appraise the caliber of quality-of-life assessments used to evaluate children, adolescents, and adults with congenital heart disease. In our appraisal, we used the criteria of Gill and Feinstein.[10] By checking the conceptual and methodological rigor of the methods used in these studies, we can provide a basis to evaluate how quality-of-life research can be interpreted and, if necessary, strengthened.

METHODS

Search strategy
We performed a PubMed search for studies that examined the quality of life in patients with congenital heart disease. We included in this review all empirical studies that assessed children, adolescents, and adults; were published in English, French, German, or Dutch; and appeared in print between January 1980 and October 2003. The search terms used were *quality of life* combined with *congenital heart, heart defects*, or terms referring to specific heart lesions (ie, *Fallot, transposition, coarctation, Eisenmenger, septal defect, atrial septal defect, ventricular septal defect, congenital aortic stenosis, congenital pulmonary stenosis, univentricular, anomalous pulmonary venous, truncus arteriosus, ductus arteriosus, Fontan, Marfan, double outlet, double inlet, Ebstein*). We excluded letters, editorials, reviews, case studies, opinion articles, studies on parents of children with congenital heart disorders, transplant-related investigations, and qualitative studies. Textbooks, proceedings, and conference abstracts were not reviewed.

Review criteria and procedure
Gill and Feinstein[10] were mainly interested in the face validity of quality-of-life measures. Hence, they evaluated the extent to which quality-of-life assessments measured the phenomenon on face value. However, before quality-of-life measurements can be evaluated, quality of life must be defined. Gill and Feinstein therefore defined quality of life as follows: "Rather than being a description of patients' health status, quality of life is a reflection of the way that patients perceive and react to their health status and to other, nonmedical aspects of their lives."[10(p619)] Using this definition, they developed 10 criteria to be used to evaluate the caliber of quality-of-life measurements. These 10 criteria follow.

1. Did the investigators give a definition of quality of life? (15% of studies adhered to this criteria.)

Because a uniform definition of quality of life presently does not exist, investigators need to clarify their conceptualization of *quality of life* to ensure that readers have a good understanding of the term as they define it. Therefore, investigators must provide an explicit definition of quality of life that serves as a basis for selecting the instruments to be used in their study. Simply referring to the wide variety of definitions, describing the components of quality of life, or citing multiple definitions without unequivocally quoting the definition underpinning the measurement is inadequate.

2. Did the investigators state the domains they will measure as components of quality of life? (47% of studies adhered to this criteria.)

Quality of life is typically considered to be a multidimensional construct, comprising multiple domains. The choice of quality-of-life instrument(s) basically relies on the components included in the instrument(s). To determine whether the selected measurement suitably represents the desired target, investigators ought to stipulate explicitly which domains they consider to be significant constituents of quality of life. Just describing domains underlying a specific questionnaire is not sufficient.

3. Did the investigators give reasons for choosing the instruments they used? (36% of studies adhered to this criteria.)

Valid assessments require that the instruments used are suitable for the intended task. Since numerous quality-of-life instruments exist, investigators need to state their reasons for choosing to use a particular instrument or instruments to assess quality of life. These reasons should ensure that quality of life will be measured appropriately according to their intended goals. Just because an instrument has good psychometric properties or is widely used does not mean suitable reasons were considered for its use.

4. Did the investigators aggregate results from multiple items, domains, or instruments into a single composite score for quality of life? (14% of studies adhered to this criteria.)

Gill and Feinstein[10] argued that an effective characterization of quality of life is enhanced if investigators present a composite score that summarizes the results of multiple items, domains, or instruments. Although the richness of a profile description may be lost, an aggregated score simplifies the communication of results and permits the assessment of interrelationship between quality of life and other variables.

5. Were patients asked to give their own global rating for quality of life? (17% of studies adhered to this criteria.)

Although quality of life is principally conceptualized as a multidimensional construct, a single global rating by the patient is useful. Patients' rating of their quality of life on a 1-item scale reflects the disparate values and preferences of individual patients.[10] Hence, such a rating serves as an overall estimate of quality of life that considers quality-of-life components deemed important by the respondent.

6. Was overall quality of life distinguished from health-related quality of life? (No studies adhered to this criteria.)

Health care professionals are predominantly interested in health-related factors to be components of patients' quality of life. However, a holistic approach implies that also nonmedical phenomena emerge, such as family relationships, social networks, spirituality, pet ownership, etc. Consequently, a distinction between overall and health-related quality of life should be made clear in quality-of-life articles. In this review, we considered this criterion to be fulfilled if the authors explicitly stated the difference between overall and health-related quality of life.

7. Were patients invited to supplement the items listed in the instruments offered by the investigators that they considered relevant for their quality of life? (13% of studies adhered to this criteria.)

Since there is a growing awareness that quality of life can only be affected by components that are important for an individual,[11] an adequate measurement of quality of life should provide the possibility for respondents to indicate the domains that are important for their quality of life. Some argue that this approach is the only way that can lead to a valid measurement of quality of life because it explicitly includes the domains that are relevant for respondents.[10,12]

8. If so, were these supplemental items incorporated into the final rating? (89% of studies adhered to this criteria.)

To take the supplemental items into consideration in the assessment of quality of life, they ought to be incorporated into the final rating. If there is no possibility of obtaining supplemental items, this criterion is not applicable.

9. Were patients allowed to indicate which items were personally important to them? (8.5% of studies adhered to this criteria.)

Patients need to have the opportunity to rate the importance of different items, either those specified by the investigators or added by the patients. This offers the possibility to individually weigh the items and precludes the assumption that all items have the same importance for all patients.

10. If so, were the importance ratings incorporated into the final rating? (50% of studies adhered to this criteria.)

As for the supplemental items, the importance rating should be incorporated into the final rating. Again, if there is no possibility of scoring the importance of different items, this criterion is not applicable.

Data analysis
For each criterion, the number of articles complying with that criterion was counted and the percentage was calculated. To indicate how well individual articles performed on the respective criteria, a summary score was calculated by summing the number of criteria an article fulfilled and dividing this sum by the number of criteria for which the article was eligible to be evaluated; the resulting value was then multiplied by 100.[10] Summary scores could range from 0, for articles complying with none of the criteria, to 100, for articles complying with all of the criteria.

Characteristics of selected articles
We identified 70 articles that met the inclusion criteria.[7-9,13-79] A total of 8206 patients were surveyed in these studies, ranging from a study sample of 9[33] to 1566 patients in the Second Natural History Study.[26] Twenty-four studies were performed in children [8,15,16,18,19,23,28,29,31,33,35,37,39, 41,42,47,48,55,60,61,68,70,72,77], 34 in adults [7,14,17,20,22,26,32,34,38,43-46,50-54,57-59,62-67,69,71,73,75,76,78,79], and 12 in a mixed population of children, adolescents, and adults.[9,13,21,24,25,27,30,36,40,49,56,74] Most investigations were conducted using patients diagnosed with tetralogy of Fallot (11 studies) [7,14,22,28,40,44,46,51,67,73,75], transposition of the great arteries (11 studies) [8,19,23,29,30,33,45,57,68,74,76], or a mix of various heart defects (11 studies). [18,31,32,34,38,47,54,64,72,77,79] The most prevalent types of patients studied were patients with more than 1 cardiac anomaly (n=1453) or those with transposed arteries (n=1117), ventricular septal defect (n=1069), a right ventricle to pulmonary artery conduit (n=910), or tetralogy of Fallot (n=868) **(Figure 1)**. Together, these patients composed more than 65% of the patients studied. Sixty-four percent of the studies were performed in the United States (n=16) [9,17,19,21,23,26,27,35,40,42,52,55,56,64,70,72], Japan (n=10) [7,13,33,37,46,49,62,66,78,79], the United Kingdom (n=7) [38,39,53,57,65,73,74], Germany (n=7) [22,28,29,32,60,61,71], and the Netherlands (n=6).[15,34,43-45,54]

Figure 1: Primary diagnosis of subjects in quality-of-life studies of congenital heart disease

[Pie chart showing segments labeled: interrupted aorta, coarctation of aorta, AVSD, TAPVU, hypoplastic left heart syndrome, Fontan, Marfan, Eisenmenger, ASD, univentricular heart, aortic valve disease, aortic valve stenosis, pulmonary valve stenosis, Fallot, RV-AP conduit, VSD, transposition, mix, pulmonary hypertension, ductus arteriosus, pulmonary atresia, Ebstein]

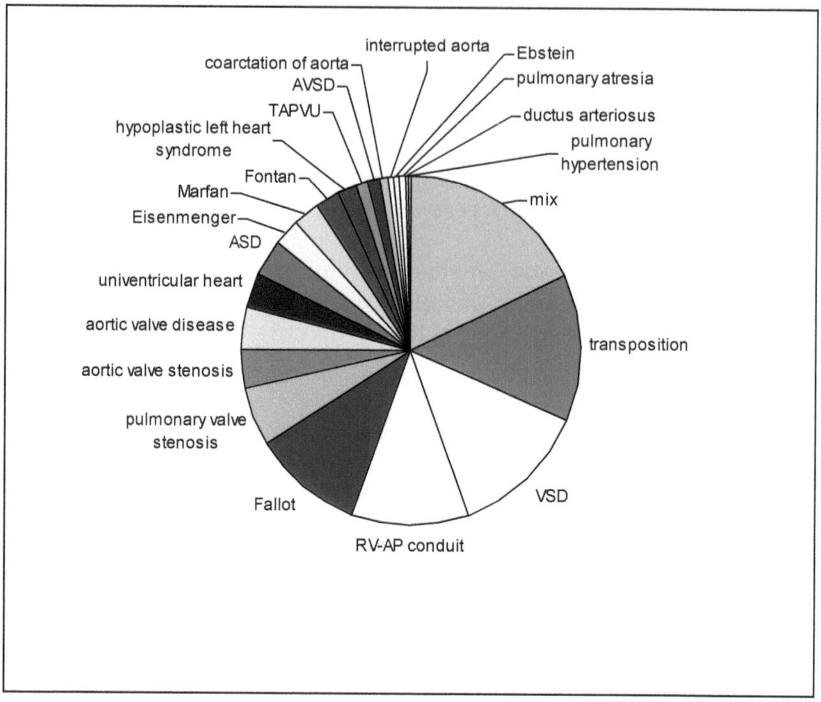

Results

The studies included in this review were selected because they all drew conclusions about patients' quality of life. However, only 53 (76%) of 70 articles explicitly aimed to measure quality of life. The other 17 articles measured a range of variables, instead of quality of life per se, but drew conclusions in terms of quality of life. Moreover, 30 articles (43%) did not describe quality of life in the Methods or Results section but merely mentioned it in the Abstract or Discussion.

Our evaluation of the rigor of quality-of-life studies in patients with congenital heart disease revealed that only 1 study (1%) provided a definition of quality of life (**Table 1**). Seventeen studies (24%) stated explicitly the domains that constitute quality of life. Two studies (3%) argued why the specific measurement was chosen. Twenty-two studies

Table 1. Evaluation of the caliber of quality-of-life assessments in congenital heart disease

First author, year of publication	Conceptual definition of QoL	Domains of QoL defined	Reason for choosing measurement	Score aggregated into a single index	Patient's rating on overall QoL	Distinction between overall and health-related QoL	Patient could supplement items	These items were incorporated in final rating	Patients could rate personal importance of items	Importance rate was incorporated into final rating	Summary score
Aeba, 2000	–	–	–	–	–	–	–	n.a.	–	n.a.	0
Aigueperse, 1991	–	–	–	–	–	–	–	n.a.	–	n.a.	0
Belli, 1999	–	–	–	–	–	–	–	n.a.	–	n.a.	0
Benatar, 1995	–	–	–	+	–	–	n.a.	n.a.	n.a.	n.a.	17
Brunet, 1986	–	–	–	–	–	–	–	n.a.	–	n.a.	0
Burkhart, 2003	–	–	–	+	–	–	n.a.	n.a.	n.a.	n.a.	17
Casey, 1994	–	–	–	–	–	–	–	n.a.	–	n.a.	0
Culbert, 2003	–	+	+	–	–	–	–	n.a.	–	n.a.	25
Daliento, 1998	–	–	–	–	–	–	–	n.a.	–	n.a.	0
Dearani, 2003	–	–	–	–	–	–	–	n.a.	–	n.a.	0
Dittrich, 1999	–	–	–	–	–	–	–	n.a.	–	n.a.	0
Dunbar-Masterson, 2001	–	–	–	–	–	–	–	n.a.	–	n.a.	0
Elkins, 1997	–	–	–	–	–	–	–	n.a.	–	n.a.	13
Fesslova, 1991	–	–	–	+	–	–	–	n.a.	–	n.a.	13
Fiane, 1996	–	–	–	–	–	–	–	n.a.	–	n.a.	0
Gersony, 1993	–	+	–	–	–	–	–	n.a.	–	n.a.	13
Haas, 2000	–	–	–	+	–	–	n.a.	n.a.	n.a.	n.a.	17
Horstkotte, 1993	–	+	–	–	–	–	–	n.a.	–	n.a.	13
Hovels-Gurich, 2002	–	+	–	–	–	–	–	n.a.	–	n.a.	13
Hucin, 2000	–	–	–	+	–	–	n.a.	n.a.	n.a.	n.a.	17
Immer, 1994	–	–	–	–	–	–	–	n.a.	–	n.a.	0
Immer, 1998	–	+	–	+	+	–	n.a.	n.a.	n.a.	n.a.	50
Ishizawa, 1985	–	–	–	–	–	–	–	n.a.	–	n.a.	0
Kamphuis, 2002	–	+	+	–	–	+	–	n.a.	+	+	56
Kirshbom, 2002	–	–	–	–	–	–	–	n.a.	–	n.a.	0
Kupilik, 1999	–	–	–	+	–	–	n.a.	n.a.	n.a.	n.a.	17
Kuribayashi, 1994	–	–	–	–	–	–	–	n.a.	–	n.a.	0
Lane, 2002	–	+	–	–	–	–	–	n.a.	–	n.a.	13
Leonard, 2000	–	–	–	+	–	–	n.a.	n.a.	n.a.	n.a.	17
Lillehei, 1986	–	+	–	–	–	–	–	n.a.	–	n.a.	13
Lozano, 1990	–	–	–	–	–	–	–	n.a.	–	n.a.	0
Mahle, 2000	–	–	–	–	–	–	–	n.a.	–	n.a.	0
Meijboom, 1994	–	–	–	+	–	–	n.a.	n.a.	n.a.	n.a.	17
Meijboom, 1995	–	–	–	+	–	–	n.a.	n.a.	n.a.	n.a.	17
Meijboom, 1996	–	–	–	+	–	–	n.a.	n.a.	n.a.	n.a.	17
Miyamura, 1993	–	–	–	–	–	–	–	n.a.	–	n.a.	0
Miyamura, 1996	–	+	–	–	–	–	–	n.a.	–	n.a.	13
Moyen Laane, 1997	–	+	–	+	–	–	–	n.a.	–	n.a.	25
Moyen Laane, 1997	–	+	–	+	–	–	–	n.a.	–	n.a.	25
Park, 1994	–	+	–	–	–	–	–	n.a.	–	n.a.	13
Peters, 2002	–	+	–	+	–	–	–	n.a.	+	+	44
Presbitero, 1988	–	–	–	+	–	–	n.a.	n.a.	n.a.	n.a.	17
Pressley, 1992	–	–	–	–	–	–	–	n.a.	–	n.a.	0
Raj Behl, 1984	–	–	–	+	–	–	n.a.	n.a.	n.a.	n.a.	17

Study	C1	C2	C3	C4	C5	C6	C7	C8	C9	C10	Score
Rietveld, 2002	−	+	−	−	−	−	−	n.a.	−	n.a.	13
Rogers, 1995	−	−	−	−	−	−	−	n.a.	−	n.a.	0
Rosenzweig, 1999	−	−	−	−	−	−	−	n.a.	−	n.a.	0
Sagin-Saylam, 1996	−	−	−	+	−	−	n.a.	n.a.	n.a.	n.a.	17
Saliba, 2001	−	−	−	−	−	−	−	n.a.	−	n.a.	0
Sandoval, 2001	−	−	−	−	−	−	−	n.a.	−	n.a.	0
Schmid, 1999	−	−	−	−	−	−	−	n.a.	−	n.a.	0
Schreiber, 1997	−	−	−	+	−	−	n.a.	n.a.	n.a.	n.a.	17
Shibata, 1996	−	−	−	+	−	−	n.a.	n.a.	n.a.	n.a.	17
Shyamkrisnan, 1996	−	−	−	−	−	−	−	n.a.	−	n.a.	0
Simko, 2003	+	+	−	+	−	−	−	n.a.	−	n.a.	38
Stewart, 1993	−	−	−	−	−	−	−	n.a.	−	n.a.	0
Sugimoto, 2001	−	−	−	−	−	−	−	n.a.	−	n.a.	0
Ternestedt, 2001	−	+	−	−	−	−	−	n.a.	−	n.a.	13
Turina, 1989	−	−	−	−	−	−	−	n.a.	−	n.a.	0
Verbraecken, 2001	−	−	−	−	−	−	−	n.a.	−	n.a.	0
Vergesslich, 1984	−	−	−	+	−	−	n.a.	n.a.	n.a.	n.a.	17
Vogel, 1999	−	−	−	+	−	−	n.a.	n.a.	n.a.	n.a.	17
Walker, 2002	−	+	−	−	−	−	−	n.a.	−	n.a.	13
Walker, 2003	−	−	−	−	−	−	−	n.a.	−	n.a.	0
Warnes, 1986	−	−	−	−	−	−	−	n.a.	−	n.a.	0
Wennevold, 1982	−	−	−	−	−	−	−	n.a.	−	n.a.	0
Wilson, 1998	−	−	−	−	−	−	−	n.a.	−	n.a.	0
Wimmer, 1990	−	−	−	−	−	−	−	n.a.	−	n.a.	0
Yamashita, 2002	−	−	−	−	−	−	−	n.a.	−	n.a.	0
Yozu, 2001	−	−	−	−	−	−	−	n.a.	−	n.a.	0
Summary of data	1%	24%	3%	31%	1%	1%	0%	n.a.	4%	100%	

(31%) assessed quality of life with a single-item instrument or with a composite score of multiple-item tools that provided 1 overall score. Only 1 study (1%) allowed the patients to self-rate their perceived quality of life. Another study (1%) explicitly distinguished between overall quality of life and health-related quality of life. In the 53 studies that used multiple-item instruments, none provided a way for the respondents to select supplemental items important to them. However, 2 studies (4%) used an instrument that allowed respondents to rate the importance of respective items in the instrument. In these 2 studies, the importance rates were incorporated into the overall score.

Summary scores for individual articles ranged from 0 to 56, with a median score of 0 (quartile 1=0; quartile 3=17). Indeed, more than half of the articles (51.4%) did not comply with any of the 10 criteria. Only 2 articles[32,34] had a summary score of 50 or higher. Across the 70 quality-of-life studies that we reviewed, 39 different tools, questionnaires, or variables were used to measure quality of life (**Table 2**). Quality of life was mostly assessed by using the New York Heart Association Classification,[80] by employment status, and by educational level. Most variables that were used referred to physical functioning, health status, or socioeconomic factors.

Table 2. Measures or variables used by authors to assess quality of life in congenital heart disease

Measures	Categories	Number of studies
NYHA functional class	Functional abilities	19
Employment	Social functioning	13
Education	Social functioning	11
Symptoms	Clinical variables	9
Pregnancies and childbearing ability	Functional abilities	8
Perceived health status (1 item)	Perceived health status	7
Marital state	Social functioning	6
Medication intake	Clinical variables	4
Ability index	Functional abilities	3
Sport and recreation	Functional abilities	3
Insurance	Social functioning	3
Neurological functioning	Clinical variables	3
Medical Outcome Study Short Form-36 (SF-36)	Perceived health status	3
Child Health Questionnaire (CHQ)	Perceived health status	3
Exercise capacity	Functional abilities	3
Protocol of Kajandi / Lindstrom	Life conditions	3
Lifestyle	Physical and social functioning	2
Possession of a driver's license	Social functioning	2
Perceived quality of life (1 item)	Overall quality of life	2
Activity level	Functional abilities	2
Functional status	Functional abilities	2
6-minute walk test	Functional abilities	1
Physical fitness	Functional abilities	1
TNO/AZL Adult Quality of Life (TAAQOL)	Emotional distress with life domains	1
Need for reoperation	Clinical variables	1
Health Utility Index	Perceived health status	1
Psychological profile	Mental health	1
Nottingham Health Profile	Perceived health status	1
Inventory for the Assessment of the Quality of Life in Children and Adolescents (IQLC)	Perceived health status + Overall quality of life	1
Quality of life questionnaire for chronic lung disease	Perceived health status	1
Duke questionnaire	Perceived health status	1
Normal unrestricted life	Functional abilities	1
Hospital admissions	Health care consumption	1
Comorbidity	Clinical variables	1
Ferrans and Powers Quality of Life Index – Cardiac Version III (QLI-Cardiac III)	Satisfaction with life domains	1
Limitations to activity	Functional abilities	1
Satisfaction with operation	Consumer satisfaction	1
Resumption of work	Social functioning	1
Sickness Impact Profile	Perceived health status	1

DISCUSSION

The evaluation of quality of life has become increasingly important in children, adolescents, and adults with congenital heart disease. This may be because of the longer life expectancy of these patients, as well as the physical, psychological, and social impediments experienced by them. Quality of life is, however, an equivocal concept. It is often used as an umbrella term to cover an assortment of concepts,[93] implying that many researchers use the label *quality of life* to describe various variables, just because quality of life is in vogue.[94] Hence, quality of life is often used inappropriately. In this review, we aimed to evaluate the conceptual and methodological rigor of published quality-of-life assessments in patients with congenital heart disease, using previously developed criteria.[10]

Based on our critical appraisal of the literature, we conclude that quality-of-life assessments in patients with congenital heart disease have major conceptual and methodological drawbacks. Only 1 investigator conceptually defined quality of life. The overall failure to provide an unequivocal definition of quality of life is problematic and compromises the interpretability of past studies. The variety of measures used in these studies illustrates the different approaches used by the investigators. More specifically, we observed that 39 different measures or instruments were used as indicators of quality of life, but only a few authors gave reasons for their choice of instruments. In some studies, their choice of a specific measure seemed arbitrary because its relevance with respect to quality of life is questionable. In what sense, for instance, is the need for reoperation or hospital admission interchangeable with quality of life?

When compared with the results of Gill and Feinstein[10] published 10 years earlier, in our updated review we found the caliber of quality-of-life assessments in the congenital heart disease population to be poorer. In our study, the percentage of articles complying with the criteria was lower in 7 of 10 criteria compared with that in the Gill and Feinstein study. We found a large difference for the criterion "reason for choosing the measurement used." This discordance is owing to our stricter interpretation of this criterion. We considered good psychometric properties or widespread use of an instrument to be inadequate reasons for using it to measure quality of life, because such reasons do not guarantee that the instrument is suitable for its intended task.[10] Moreover, the validity and reliability of an instrument assessed in a particular sample and setting cannot be extrapolated to other settings or populations. Our review turned up a substantially higher proportion of studies in which an overall score was given. This is because, unlike Gill and Feinstein,[10] we considered also as an overall score the use of a single-item instrument or classification system such as the New York Heart Association Functional Class.[80] Recall, many studies we reviewed used the New York Heart Association Classification to assess quality of life in patients with congenital heart disease. Only for the criterion "incorporating importance ratings into the final quality of life score" did we find a 100% compliance. This is because the instruments used in the 2 studies that allowed respondents to rate the importance of respective items (Ferrans and Powers Quality of Life Index, cardiac version III[50];

TNO-AZL Questionnaire for Adult's Health-Related Quality of Life[34]) also included these importance scores in their final ratings.

This review confirmed that the term *quality of life* is also often used inappropriately in studies of patients with congenital heart disease. Indeed, a quarter of the articles reviewed drew conclusions about patients' quality of life, although they failed to measure it. Consequently, if health care professionals were to rely on the findings of the articles reviewed here in terms of outcome evaluation, the resulting medical decision making or health policy would be suspect. Thus, it is imperative that researchers use a more thorough conceptual and methodological basis in their quality-of-life studies. Furthermore, researchers need to be aware of the potential confusion that they may introduce if they conclude that patients have a good or bad quality of life when, in fact, they did not actually measure quality of life. This stresses the importance of designing quality-of-life studies based on a sound conceptualization and avoiding the incorrect use of the term *quality of life*.

Inspired by the results of this literature review, we conducted a thorough conceptualization of quality of life (see chapter 2). Based on existing concept analyses of quality of life published in the literature[11,95,96] and relying on the evaluation of different conceptual pitfalls, we concluded that satisfaction with life is the most suitable approach for defining quality of life. However, none of the existing definitions of quality of life, reviewed in the context of life satisfaction, explicitly integrates aspects of the conceptual pitfalls identified. Therefore, after integrating the formulated critiques, we defined quality of life as

> *the degree of overall life satisfaction that is positively or negatively influenced by an individual's perception of certain aspects of life that are important to them, including matters both related and unrelated to health.*

According to this definition, quality of life can, for instance, be measured using the Satisfaction With Life Scale.[97] This does not, however, dismiss the utility of generic and disease-specific instruments in measuring specific determinants or components of quality of life. While these instruments may not measure quality of life itself, they may be useful in measuring disability related to specific diseases and effectiveness of treatment. Such instruments augment insights in the self-perceived health status or functional abilities of the patients under study. In addition, we suggest to researchers planning to conduct quality-of-life studies to use the Gill and Feinstein[10] criteria to strengthen their methods and thus avoid current flaws.

Two possible limitations of the present study can be identified. First, the criteria used in this review were developed in the early 1990s to critically appraise the caliber of quality-of-life studies in the medical literature.[10] Whether they currently remain applicable might be questioned, because conceptual understanding of quality of life may have evolved during the last decade. Indeed, several authors have, in the meantime, published their concept analyses of quality of life.[95,96,98-103] Moreover, the equal weighting of the 10 criteria may be subject to debate. Second, we did not include all quality of life articles published, because we only reviewed articles contained in the PubMed database. Although searching other databases, such as Psychinfo, CINAHL, or Embase, may have resulted in more relevant articles, nevertheless, we believe that such searches would not have dramatically affected the conclusions of this review because we focused on conceptual and methodological issues, rather than on the findings of respective studies themselves. A specific selection bias is therefore unlikely.

CONCLUSION

Quality of life is an important issue in patients with congenital heart disease. Numerous studies have investigated or drawn conclusions about quality of life in this patient population. The poor conceptual and methodological basis used in these studies implies that many results of quality-of-life studies in patients with congenital heart disease are inconclusive. We appeal for more conceptual and methodological rigor with respect to future quality-of-life studies in this group of patients.

REFERENCES

1. Boneva RS, Botto LD, Moore CA, Yang Q, Correa A, Erickson JD. *Mortality associated with congenital heart defects in the United States: trends and racial disparities, 1979-1997.* Circulation. 2001;103:2376-2381.
2. Grech V, Savona-Ventura C. *Declining mortality from congenital heart disease related to innovations in diagnosis and treatment: a population-based study.* Cardiol Young. 1999;9:78-80.
3. McGrath KA, Truesdell SC. *Employability and career counseling for adolescents and adults with congenital heart disease.* Nurs Clin North Am. 1994; 29:319-330.
4. Hart EM, Garson A. *Psychosocial concerns of adults with congenital heart disease: employability and insurability.* Cardiol Clin. 1993;11:711-715.
5. KamphuisM, Vogels T, Ottenkamp J, Van Der Wall EE, Verloove-Vanhorick SP, Vliegen HW. *Employment in adults with congenital heart disease.* Arch Pediatr Adolesc Med. 2002;156:1143-1148.
6. Simko LC. *Adults with congenital heart disease: utilizing quality of life and Husted's nursing theory as a conceptual framework.* Crit Care Nurs Q. 1999;22:1-11.

7. Miyamura H, Eguchi S, Asano K. Long-term results of the intracardiac repair of tetralogy of Fallot: a follow-up study conducted over more than 20 years on 100 consecutive operative survivors. Surg Today. 1993;23:1049-1052.
8. Belli E, Lacour-Gayet F, Serraf A, et al. Surgical management of transposition of great arteries associated with multiple ventricular septal defects. Eur J Cardiothorac Surg. 1999;16:14-20.
9. Elkins RC, Knottcraig CJ, Mccue C, Lane MM. Congenital aortic valve disease - improved survival and quality of life. Ann Surg. 1997;225:503-510.
10. Gill TM, Feinstein AR. A critical appraisal of the quality of quality-of-life measurements. JAMA. 1994;272:619-626.
11. Ferrans CE. Development of a conceptual model of quality of life. Sch Inq Nurs Pract. 1996;10:293-304.
12. Hickey AM, Bury G, O'Boyle CA, Bradley F, O'Kelly FD, Shannon W. A new short form individual quality of life measure (SEIQoL-DW): application in a cohort of individuals with HIV/AIDS. BMJ. 1996;313:29-33.
13. Aeba R, Katogi T, Takeuchi S, Kawada S. Outcome of patients with cyanotic congenital heart disease undergoing a second systemic-to-pulmonary artery shunt. J Cardiovasc Surg (Torino). 2000;41:23-30.
14. Aigueperse J, Marechal MC. Evaluation of the quality of life in adulthood of 158 patients surgically-treated for tetralogy of Fallot [in French]. Arch Mal Coeur Vaiss. 1991;84:685-690.
15. Benatar A, Tanke R, Roef M, Meyboom EJ, Van De Wal HJ. Mid-term results of the modified Senning operation for cavopulmonary connection with autologous tissue. Eur J Cardiothorac Surg. 1995;9:320-324.
16. Brunet D, Losay J, Bruniaux J, Binet JP, Planche C, Langlois J. Long-term evolution of children with single ventricles after palliative surgery [in French]. Arch Mal Coeur Vaiss. 1986;79:107-112.
17. Burkhart HM, Dearani JA, Mair DD, et al. The modified Fontan procedure: early and late results in 132 adult patients. J Thorac Cardiovasc Surg. 2003;125: 1252-1259.
18. Casey FA, Craig BG, Mulholland HC. Quality-of-life in surgically palliated complex congenital heart-disease. Arch Dis Child. 1994;70:382-386.
19. Culbert EL, Ashburn DA, Cullen-Dean G, et al. Quality of life of children after repair of transposition of the great arteries. Circulation. 2003;108:857-862.
20. Daliento L, Somerville J, Presbitero P, et al. Eisenmenger syndrome: factors relating to deterioration and death. Eur Heart J. 1998;19:1845-1855.
21. Dearani JA, Danielson GK, Puga FJ, et al. Late follow-up of 1095 patients undergoing operation for complex congenital heart disease utilizing pulmonary ventricle to pulmonary artery conduits. Ann Thorac Surg. 2003;75:399-410.
22. Dittrich S, Vogel M, Dahnert I, Berger F, Lange PE. Surgical repair of tetralogy of Fallot in adults today. Clin Cardiol. 1999;22:460-464.
23. Dunbar-Masterson C, Wypij D, Bellinger DC, et al. General health status of children with d-transposition of the great arteries after the arterial switch operation. Circulation. 2001;104:I138-I142.
24. Fesslova V, Hunter S, Stark J, Taylor JF. The long-term clinical outcome of patients with tricuspid atresia, II: influence of surgical procedures. J Cardiovasc Surg (Torino). 1991;32:225-232.
25. Fiane AE, Lindberg HL, Saatvedt K, Svennevig JL. Mechanical valve replacement in congenital heart disease. J Heart Valve Dis. 1996;5:337-342.
26. Gersony WM, Hayes CJ, Driscoll DJ, et al. Second natural history study of congenital heart defects: quality of life of patients with aortic stenosis, pulmonary stenosis, or ventricular septal defect. Circulation. 1993;87:I52-I65.
27. Haas GS, Hess H, Black M, Onnasch J, Mohr FW, Van Son JAM. Extracardiac conduit Fontan procedure: early and intermediate results. Eur J Cardiothorac Surg. 2000;17:648-654.
28. Horstkotte D, Paselk C, Bircks W, Loogen F. Clinical long-term results after corrective surgery of tetralogy of Fallot [in German]. Z Kardiol. 1993;82:552-562.
29. Hovels-Gurich HH, Konrad K, Wiesner M, et al. Long term behavioural outcome after neonatal arterial switch operation for transposition of the great arteries. Arch Dis Child. 2002;87:506-510.

30. Hucin B, Voriskova M, Hruda J, et al. Late complications and quality of life after atrial correction of transposition of the great arteries in 12 to 18 year follow-up. J Cardiovasc Surg (Torino). 2000;41:233-239.
31. Immer FF, Haefelibleuer B, Seiler A, Stocker F, Weber JW. Congenital heartdisease - prevalence and course during compulsory schooling (8th to 16th year of life) [in German]. Schweiz Med Wochenschr. 1994;124:893-899.
32. Immer FF, Seiler AM, Stocker F. Status and after-care of young adults with congenital heart defects [in German]. Schweiz Med Wochenschr. 1998;128: 1012-1019.
33. Ishizawa E, Tadokoro M, Satoh S, et al. Mustard procedure for simple transposition of the great arteries. Tohoku J Exp Med. 1985;145:91-96.
34. Kamphuis M, Ottenkamp J, Vliegen HW, et al. Health related quality of life and health status in adult survivors with previously operated complex congenital heart disease. Heart. 2002;87:356-362.
35. Kirshbom PM, Myung RJ, Gaynor JW, et al. Preoperative pulmonary venous obstruction affects long-term outcome for survivors of total anomalous pulmonary venous connection repair. Ann Thorac Surg. 2002;74:1616-1620.
36. Kupilik N, Simon P, Moidl R, et al. Valve-preserving treatment of Ebstein's anomaly: perioperative and follow-up results. Thorac Cardiovasc Surg. 1999;47:229-234.
37. Kuribayashi R, Sekine S, Aida H, et al. Long-term results of primary closure for ventricular septal-defects in the first year of life. Surg Today. 1994;24:389-392.
38. Lane DA, Lip GY, Millane TA. Quality of life in adults with congenital heart disease. Heart. 2002;88:71-75.
39. Leonard H, Derrick G, O'Sullivan J, Wren C. Natural and unnatural history of pulmonary atresia. Heart. 2000;84:499-503.
40. Lillehei CW, Varco RL, Cohen M, et al. The first open heart corrections of tetralogy of Fallot: a 26-31 year follow-up of 106 patients. Ann Surg. 1986; 204:490-502.
41. Lozano C, Rovirosa M, Reig J, Salva JA. Surgery of atrioventricular septal-defects: review of the first 100 cases. Eur J Cardiothorac Surg. 1990;4:359-364.
42. Mahle WT, Clancy RR, Moss EM, Gerdes M, Jobes DR, Wernovsky G. Neurodevelopmental outcome and lifestyle assessment in school-aged and adolescent children with hypoplastic left heart syndrome. Pediatrics. 2000;105: 1082-1089.
43. Meijboom F, Szatmari A, Utens E, et al. Long-term follow-up after surgical closure of ventricular septal defect in infancy and childhood. J Am Coll Cardiol. 1994;24:1358-1364.
44. Meijboom F, Szatmari A, Deckers JW, et al. Cardiac status and health-related quality of life in the long term after surgical repair of tetralogy of Fallot in infancy and childhood. J Thorac Cardiovasc Surg. 1995;110:883-891.
45. Meijboom F, Szatmari A, Deckers JW, et al. Long-term follow-up (10 to 17 years) after Mustard repair for transposition of the great arteries. J Thorac Cardiovasc Surg. 1996;111:1158-1168.
46. Miyamura H, Takahashi M, Sugawara M, Eguchi S. The long-term influence of pulmonary valve regurgitation following repair of tetralogy of Fallot: does preservation of the pulmonary valve ring affect quality of life? Surg Today. 1996; 26:603-606.
47. Moyen , Laane KM, Meberg A, Otterstad JE, et al. Quality of life in children with congenital heart defects. Acta Paediatr. 1997;86:975-980.
48. Laane KM, Meberg A, Otterstad JE, Froland G, Lindstrom B, Eriksson B. Does an early neonatal diagnosis of a later spontaneously closed ventricular septal defect impair quality of life? Scand Cardiovasc J. 1997;31:213-216.
49. Park I, Nakazawa M, Imai Y, Sawatari K, Momma K. Prediction of quality of life at long-term follow-up after Fontan operation by scoring risk factors. Jpn Circ J. 1994;58:646-652.
50. Peters KF, Kong F, Hanslo M, Biesecker BB. Living with Marfan syndrome, III: quality of life and reproductive planning. Clin Genet. 2002;62:110-120.
51. Presbitero P, Demarie D, Aruta E, et al. Results of total correction of tetralogy of Fallot performed in adults. Ann Thorac Surg. 1988;46:297-301.
52. Pressley JC, Wharton JM, Tang ASL, Lowe JE, Gallagher JJ, Prystowsky EN. Effect of Ebsteins anomaly on short-term and long-term outcome of surgically treated patients with Wolff-Parkinson-White syndrome. Circulation. 1992; 86:1147-1155.
53. Raj Behl P, Blesovsky A. Ebstein's anomaly: sixteen years' experience with valve replacement without plication of the right ventricle. Thorax. 1984;39:8-13.

54. Rietveld S, Mulder BJ, Van BI, et al. Negative thoughts in adults with congenital heart disease. Int J Cardiol. 2002;86:19-26.
55. Rogers BT, Msall ME, Buck GM, et al. Neurodevelopmental outcome of infants with hypoplastic left heart syndrome. J Pediatr. 1995;126:496-498.
56. Rosenzweig EB, Kerstein D, Barst RJ. Long-term prostacyclin for pulmonary hypertension with associated congenital heart defects. Circulation. 1999; 99:1858-1865.
57. Sagin-Saylam G, Somerville J. Palliative Mustard operation for transposition of the great arteries: late results after 15-20 years. Heart. 1996;75:72-77.
58. Saliba Z, Butera G, Bonnet D, et al. Quality of life and perceived health status in surviving adults with univentricular heart. Heart. 2001;86:69-73.
59. Sandoval J, Aguirre JS, Pulido T, et al. Nocturnal oxygen therapy in patients with the Eisenmenger syndrome. Am J Respir Crit Care Med. 2001;164:1682-1687.
60. Schmid FX, Kampmann C, Peivandi AA, Oelert H. Surgical treatment of hypoplastic left heart syndrome: experience with staged palliative reconstruction [in German]. Herz. 1999;24:307-314.
61. Schreiber C, Mazzitelli D, Haehnel JC, Lorenz HP, Meisner H. The interrupted aortic arch: an overview after 20 years of surgical treatment. Eur J Cardiothorac Surg. 1997;12:466-469.
62. Shibata Y, Abe T, Kuribayashi R, et al. Surgical treatment of isolated secundum atrial septal defect in patients more than 50 years old. Ann Thorac Surg. 1996; 62:1096-1099.
63. Shyamkrishnan KG, Singh M, Tharakan JM, Dal A. A ten-year post-surgical assessment of pulmonary hypertension in adults with patent ductus arteriosus. Indian Heart J. 1996;48:249-251.
64. Simko LC, Mcginnis KA. Quality of life experienced by adults with congenital heart disease. AACN Clin Issues. 2003;14:42-53.
65. Stewart AB, Ahmed R, Travill CM, Newman CG. Coarctation of the aorta life and health 20-44 years after surgical repair. Br Heart J. 1993;69:65-70.
66. Sugimoto S, Takagi N, Hachiro Y, Abe T. High frequency of arrhythmias after Fontan operation indicates earlier anticoagulant therapy. Int J Cardiol. 2001; 78:33-39.
67. Ternestedt BM, Wall K, Oddsson H, Riesenfeld T, Groth I, Schollin J. Quality of life 20 and 30 years after surgery in patients operated on for tetralogy of Fallot and for atrial septal defect. Pediatr Cardiol. 2001;22:128-132.
68. Turina MI, Siebenmann R, Vonsegesser L, Schonbeck M, Senning A. Late functional deterioration after atrial correction for transposition of the great arteries. Circulation. 1989;80:II62-II67.
69. Verbraecken J, Declerck A, Van De Heyning P, De Backer W, Wouters EFM. Evaluation for sleep apnea in patients with Ehlers-Danlos syndrome and Marfan: a questionnaire study. Clin Genet. 2001;60:360-365.
70. Vergesslich KA, Gersony WM, Steeg CN, et al. Postoperative assessment of porcine-valved right ventricular pulmonary-artery conduits. Am J Cardiol. 1984; 53:202-205.
71. Vogel M, Berger F, Kramer A, Alexi-Meshkishvili V, Lange PE. Diagnose und chirurgische Behandlung von Vorhofseptumdefekten im Erwachsenenalter. Dtsch Med Wochenschr. 1999;124:35-38.
72. Walker RE, Gauvreau K, Jenkins KJ. Health-related quality of life in children attending a cardiology clinic. Pediatr Cardiol. 2004;25:40-48.
73. Walker WT, Temple IK, Gnanapragasam JP, Goddard JR, Brown EM. Quality of life after repair of tetralogy of Fallot. Cardiol Young. 2002;12:549-553.
74. Warnes CA, Somerville J. Tricuspid atresia in adolescents and adults: current state and late complications. Br Heart J. 1986;56:535-543.
75. Wennevold A, Rygg I, Lauridsen P, Efsen F, Jacobsen JR. Fourteen- to nineteen year follow-up after corrective repair for tetralogy of Fallot. Scand J Thorac Cardiovasc Surg. 1982;16:41-45.
76. Wilson NJ, Clarkson PM, Barratt-Boyes BG, et al. Long-term outcome after the Mustard repair for simple transposition of the great arteries: 28-year follow-up. J Am Coll Cardiol. 1998;32:758-765.
77. Wimmer M, Salzer U, Schlemmer M, Marx M, Proll E. Experience with longterm nifedipine therapy in paediatric cardiological patients. Padiatr Padol. 1990; 25:181-193.

78. Yamashita K, Kazui T, Terada H, et al. Total and subtotal aortic replacement for extensive aortic dissection in patients with or without Marfan's syndrome. Jpn J Thorac Cardiovasc Surg. 2002;50:315-320.
79. Yozu R, Shin H, Maehara T, Iino Y, Mitsumaru A, Kawada S. Port-access cardiac surgery: experience with 34 cases at Keio University Hospital. Jpn J Thorac Cardiovasc Surg. 2001;49:360-364.
80. The Criteria Committee of the New York Heart Association. Nomenclature and Criteria for Diagnosis of Diseases of the Heart and Great Vessels. 9th ed. Boston, Mass: Little, Brown and Co; 1994:253-256.
81. Somerville J. 'Grown-up' survivors of congenital heart disease: who knows? who cares? Br J Hosp Med. 1990;43:132-136.
82. Ware JE Jr, Snow KK, Kosinski M, Gandek B. SF-36 Health Survey: Manual and Interpretation Guide. Boston, Mass: the Health Institute, New England Medical Center; 1993.
83. Landgraf JM, Abetz L, Ware JE. The CHQ User's Manual. 2nd ed. Boston, Mass: HealthAct; 1999.
84. Lindström B. The Essence of Existence: On the Quality of Life of Children in the Nordic Countries. Göteborg, Sweden: The Nordic School of Public Health; 1994.
85. Fekkes M, Kamphius RP, Ottenkamp J, et al. Health-related quality of life in young adults with minor congenital heart disease. Psychol Health. 2001;16:239-251.
86. Feeny D, Furlong W, Barr RD. Multiattributable approach to the assessment of health-related quality of life: Health Utilities Index. Med Pediatr Oncol. 1998; (suppl 1):54-59.
87. Hunt SM, McKenna SP, McEwen J, Williams J, Papp E. The Nottingham Health Profile: subjective health status and medical consultations. Soc Sci Med [A]. 1981;15:221-229.
88. Mattejat F, Jungmann J, Meusers M, et al. An inventory for assessing the qualityof life of children and adolescents: a pilot study. Z Kinder Jugendpsychiatr Psychother. 1998;26:174-182.
89. Guyatt GH, Berman LB, Townsend M, Pugsley SO, Chambers LW. A measure of quality of life for clinical trials in chronic lung disease. Thorax. 1987;42: 773-778.
90. Parkerson GR Jr, Broadhead WE, Tse CK. The Duke Health Profile: a 17-item measure of health and dysfunction. Med Care. 1990;28:1056-1072.
91. Ferrans CE, Powers MJ. Quality of Life Index: development and psychometric properties. ANS Adv Nurs Sci. 1985;8:15-24.
92. Bergner M, Bobbitt RA, Kressel S, Pollard WE, Gilson BS, Morris JR. The Sickness Impact Profile: conceptual formulation and methodology for the development of a health status measure. Int J Health Serv. 1976;6:393-415.
93. Feinstein AR. Clinimetric perspectives. J Chronic Dis. 1987;40:635-640.
94. Kinney MR. Quality of life research: rigor or rigor mortis. Cardiovasc Nurs. 1995; 31:25-28.
95. Meeberg GA. Quality of life: a concept analysis. J Adv Nurs. 1993;18:32-38.
96. Zhan L. Quality of life: conceptual and measurement issues. J Adv Nurs. 1992; 17:795-800.
97. Diener E, Emmons RA, Larsen RJ, Griffin S. The Satisfaction With Life Scale. J Pers Assess. 1985;49:71-75.
98. Felce D. Defining and applying the concept of quality of life. J Intellect Disabil Res. 1997;41:126-135.
99. Ferrans CE. Quality of life: conceptual issues. Semin Oncol Nurs. 1990;6:248-254.
100. Haas BK. A multidisciplinary concept analysis of quality of life. West J Nurs Res. 1999;21:728-742.
101. Haas BK. Clarification and integration of similar quality of life concepts. Image J Nurs Sch. 1999;31:215-220.
102. Stewart AL. Conceptual and methodologic issues in defining quality of life: state of the art. Prog Cardiovasc Nurs. 1992;7:3-11.
103. Kleinpell RM. Concept analysis of quality of life. Dimens Crit Care Nurs. 1991; 10:223-229.

Chapter 2

Quality of life: what is it and what is being measured?

Quality of life is an increasingly popular concept in the field of nursing and medicine. Since the 1970s, the number of articles on quality of life appearing in the biomedical literature has increased exponentially.[1] As of 2006, more than 10,000 articles referring to 'quality of life' are published annually. There are two possible explanations for the increasing interest in quality of life in health care. One explanation is an increased life expectancy resulting from improved medical therapies. As a result, many more individuals are diagnosed with chronic, clinically manageable illnesses, which intrude on patient's life. Hence, in addition to mortality and morbidity, quality of life must also be used to assess health care outcomes.[2] A second explanation is the abundance of medical and surgical technologies. The increase in available treatments, often with comparable effects, necessitates thorough consideration of the benefit-burden ratio of equivalent therapies. In particular, a substantial number of drugs and interventions comparably affect the outcome of disease in terms of patient survival and/or morbidity. Quality of life issues are then included in the assessment of the benefits of different treatment options.

Despite the increasing interest in quality of life, consensus is lacking on the definition of quality of life. Quality of life is often used as a generic label to describe an assortment of physical and psychosocial variables. Therefore, quality of life often seems to be an umbrella term,[3] covering a variety of concepts, such as functioning, health status, perceptions, life conditions, behaviour, happiness, lifestyle, symptoms, etc.[4] The absence of a uniform definition makes quality of life to be an ambiguous concept. The aim of the present article is to briefly describe different conceptualizations of quality of life, to evaluate the appropriateness of the respective conceptualisations, and finally to describe the consequences for the measurement of quality of life.

CONCEPTUALIZATIONS OF QUALITY OF LIFE

A spectrum of definitions of quality of life has been described in the literature. In the early 1990s, Ferrans developed a useful taxonomy of the conceptualizations of quality of life,[5-7] grouping them into six broad categories: normal life; social utility; happiness/affect; satisfaction with life; achievement of personal goals; and natural capacities. More recently, we added two other conceptualizations: utility and satisfaction with specific life domains.[1]

Normal life – Normal life is defined as the ability to supply basic needs and to maintain health and well-being.[8] Alternatively, it is defined as the absence of limitations in functional abilities, mental status, and prolonged life.[9] In this respect, quality of life is considered to be a broad concept that primarily focuses on whether disease or impairment limits a person's ability to fulfil a normal role.[10] The conceptualisation of quality of life in terms of a normal life compares the functioning of the respondent with that of healthy persons or modal individuals of the same age group.[11]

Social utility – Social utility defines quality of life according to one's ability to lead a socially "useful" life.[12] This definition considers a patient's ability to make meaningful contributions to society through gainful employment or by fulfilling socially valued roles, such as that of a teacher, volunteer, parent, etc.[6]

Utility –Utility refers to preference-based health state valuations. This is frequently used in cost evaluations in health care. Utility measures provide a quantitative estimate of preferences for particular health states, primarily obtained from a representative sample of the general population. For each health state a corresponding index value ranging from 0 to 1 is computed. An index of 0 corresponds to death while that of 1 corresponds to perfect health.[13]

Happiness/Affect – This conceptualisation of quality of life focuses on the emotional status of the respondent and reflects his/her feelings at that moment. Happiness/affect concerns the balance between positive feelings (elation) and negative feelings (depression).[6] It is a temporary and sometimes short-term affective state that is influenced by many external and internal factors.

Satisfaction with life - Satisfaction with life is the degree to which a person positively evaluates the overall quality of his/her life.[14] It refers to the level of enjoyment and contentment with the life led so far.[14]

Satisfaction with specific domains – This conceptualization refers to the satisfaction one experiences in various domains of life, such as love, marriage, friendship, leisure, job, etc.[6;15] The level of satisfaction with specific domains can range from deprivation to fulfilment.[6]

Achievement of personal goals – With this conceptualisation, quality of life is expressed in terms of the discrepancy between an individual's actual status and what he/she desires or expects.[16] This difference between expectations and actual experiences is referred to as Calman's gap.[17] The concept of achievement of personal goals assumes that quality of life is enhanced if an individual can accomplish his/her goals.

Natural capacity – Quality of life viewed in terms of natural capacity encompasses the presence of normally inborn physical and mental capabilities, both actual and potential. Natural capacity deals with very fundamental needs: for instance, relief of severe pain or being able to interact with the environment. Definitions of quality of life in terms of natural capacity are primarily developed for ethical debates and for cases in which the condition of a patient or an unborn child is such that health care professionals are asked to end life.[18] Quality of life, from this perspective, is used to provide an answer to the question: Is this a life worth living?

CONCEPTUAL ISSUES TO QUALITY OF LIFE

The diversity of approaches to defining quality of life compels to make a critical appraisal of the value of the various quality of life conceptualisations by analyzing the limitations of each approach. In 1995, Kinney described several conceptual problems.[19] Through a review of the biomedical, psychological, and social sciences literature, we elaborated on the Kinney critiques and described six conceptual problems inherent to the notion of quality of life: i) quality of life must not be used interchangeably with health status or functional abilities; ii) quality of life relies on a subjective appraisal, rather than on objective parameters; iii) there is a poor distinction between indicators and determinants of quality of life; iv) quality of life can change over time, but does not fluctuate greatly; v) quality of life can be positively or negatively influenced; vi) assessment of overall quality of life is preferred over health-related quality of life. These conceptual problems are extensively described elsewhere.[1;20]

CONCEPTUAL DEFINITION OF QUALITY OF LIFE

To assess the appropriateness of the different conceptualizations of quality of life, we evaluated them on the basis of the conceptual problems described in the previous paragraph. This revealed that only the conceptualization in terms of life satisfaction deals with all the conceptual problems.[1] Consequently, life satisfaction is the most suitable approach to define quality of life. This corresponds with the majority of concept analyses of quality of life published in the literature,[5;7;21] as well as with the results of a study using structural equation modeling.[22]

Reviewing the existing definitions of quality of life as satisfaction with life, none of them have explicitly integrated aspects of the conceptual problems. Therefore, it was suggested to include, adapt or merge components of existing definitions, integrating the formulated critiques, in order to construct a sound conceptual definition of quality of life. Accordingly, quality of life could be conceptually defined as *"the degree of overall life satisfaction that is positively or negatively influenced by an individual's perception of certain aspects of life that are important to them, including matters both related and unrelated to health"*.[23]

This definition precludes that quality of life is interchanged with health status or functional status, as it refers to a general life satisfaction. It also stresses the subjective approach of quality of life, in which individuals' perceptions are essential in the assessment. Furthermore, the definition suggests that the only indicator of quality of life is the feeling of overall life satisfaction, whereas other variables are determinants with a positive or negative impact. In this respect, quality of life could be assumed to be a unidimensional construct, though it is influenced by multiple factors (multifactorial). Quality of life is not limited to health-related issues, but includes also non-medical aspects. Because the relative importance of the respective determinants may vary over time, quality of life is precluded to be a static trait.

APPROACHES IN THE MEASUREMENT OF QUALITY OF LIFE

There are two major approaches for measuring quality of life: the "need approach" and the "want approach".[24] According to the need approach, quality of life depends on fulfillment of basic needs, such as good health, sufficient mobility, good physical performance, adequate nutrition, and favorable shelter. In this approach, quality of life is measured using standardized and predefined questionnaires about components or determinants of quality of life. Three types of measures are often used in this respect: 1) generic instruments, which comprehensively assess quality of life in a variety of populations; 2) disease-specific instruments, which are developed for a particular disease or health condition; and 3) test batteries, which employ both generic and disease-specific instruments.[25]

About 15 years ago, the use of standard tools for measuring quality of life began to be criticized for several reasons. First, such predetermined tools contain items that may not be relevant for all individuals whose quality of life is assessed.[26] Even when tools are constructed based on data from in-depth interviews with experienced patients, they do not represent the perspective of all patients. Second, standardized tools assume that all aspects applied are of equal importance for all respondents,[26] neglecting the variation of importance of different life areas for individual subjects.[27] Third, quality of life questionnaires are mostly focused on limitations and impediments, without considering positive elements that contribute to the quality of life.[28] Measurement of quality of life should therefore include the possibility that quality of life can be evaluated both in positive and negative terms.

Because of these critiques, the want approach has been developed. The want approach assumes that quality of life can only be affected by factors important to an individual.[24] For example, according to the want approach, quality of life depends on lifestyle, previous experiences, ambitions, and dreams.[24] Hence, in this approach, quality of life must be measured with instruments that permit respondents to indicate and respectively rate domains that are specifically important for *their* quality of life (i.e., individual quality of life). During the last decade, a paradigm shift has taken place in the measurement of quality of life, from one based on the need approach to one based on the want approach. Some now argue that the want approach is the most valid way of measuring quality of life, because it explicitly includes domains that are relevant for the respondents.[27;29] This is obviously a limitation of the need approach.

INSTRUMENTS TO MEASURE QUALITY OF LIFE

When researchers choose particular instruments to measure quality of life in their studies, they ought to make sure that they have a sound conceptual basis to rely on. The conceptual definition proposed in this article suggests that quality of life is a unidimensional (indicator), but multifactorial construct (determinants). Hence, we need to distinguish between instruments measuring indicators of quality of life and instruments measuring determinants of quality of life.

Indicators
Two examples of instruments that measure indicators of quality of life are a Linear Analog Scale (LAS) and the Satisfaction with Life Scale (SWLS). A LAS consist, for instance, of a vertically oriented, graded, 10-centimeter line, ranging from 0 (worst imaginable quality of life) to 100 (best imaginable quality of life). Respondents are asked to rating their overall quality of life by marking whichever point on the scale that indicates how good or bad their quality of life is in their opinion.

The SWLS consists of five statements referring to general life satisfaction.[30] Responses are scored on a 7-point Likert scale, ranging from 1 (strongly disagree) to 7 (strongly agree). An overall score can be computed by summing the individual item scores, with the minimum possible score being 5 and the maximum score 35.

Psychometric properties of both instruments have been investigated in various patient populations. These studies indicate that both the LAS and the SWLS have high content validity and a moderate to high stability.[30;31] The SWLS seems to have an internal consistency ranging from 0.80 to 0.89.[30;32] Hence, these instruments can be considered as valid and reliable for their purpose.

Determinants
Determinants of quality of life can, for instance, be measured using the 'Schedule for the Evaluation of Individual Quality of Life' (SEIQoL)[33] or its short form: the 'Schedule for the Evaluation of Individual Quality of Life – Direct Weighting' (SEIQoL-DW).[27;34] The SEIQoL and SEIQol-DW consists of three successive steps. Patients are asked 1) to name the five most important domains for their quality of life, 2) to rate the actual status on each domain, and 3) to indicate the relative weighting of each domain. In the SEIQoL, the third step is done by a judgement analysis of a series of presented cases, while in the SEIQoL-DW, patients can quantify the relative importance of each nominated domain using a colored 5-segment disk. The SEIQoL and SEIQoL-DW were created to measure individual quality of life. From this perspective, it is argued that both instruments have high face and content validity.[2;26;27;34;35] However, in a study conducted in patients with congenital heart disease, we found that this instrument measures determinants of quality of life, rather than quality of life itself.[36] That study confirmed that the SEIQoL-DW is valid and reliable to measure determinants of quality of life.[36] Since it provides the possibility to respondents to indicate the domains that are important for their quality of life, and to subsequently rate how important the respective domains are, the SEIQoL and SEIQoL-DW fits into the want approach.

Conclusion

Quality of life is a popular concept, of which the use in biomedical literature is continuously growing. Although different conceptualizations of quality of life exist, the most appropriate conceptualization appears to define quality of life in terms of life satisfaction. Researchers should rely on such conceptual foundations in order to choose the most suitable instruments for measuring quality of life. Examples of appropriate instruments to measure indicators of quality of life are a Linear Analog Scale or the Satisfaction with Life Scale. Determinants of quality of life can be measured using the Schedule for the Evaluation of Individual Quality of Life – Direct Weighting.

Reference

1. Moons P, Budts W, De Geest S. Critique on the conceptualisation of quality of life: A review and evaluation of different conceptual approaches. Int J Nurs Stud 2006; 43(7):891-901.
2. Macduff C. Respondent-generated quality of life measures: useful tools for nursing or more fool's gold? J Adv Nurs 2000; 32(2):375-382.
3. Feinstein AR. Clinimetric perspectives. J Chronic Dis 1987; 40(6):635-640.
4. Simko LC. Adults with congenital heart disease: utilizing quality of life and Husted's nursing theory as a conceptual framework. Crit Care Nurs Q 1999; 22(3):1-11.
5. Ferrans CE. Quality of life: conceptual issues. Semin Oncol Nurs 1990; 6(4):248-254.
6. Ferrans CE. Conceptualizations of quality of life in cardiovascular research. Prog Cardiovasc Nurs 1992; 7(1):2-6.
7. Ferrans CE. Development of a conceptual model of quality of life. Sch Inq Nurs Pract 1996; 10(3):293-304.
8. Leidy NK. Functional status and the forward progress of merry-go-rounds: Toward a coherent analytical framework. Nursing Research 1994; 43(4):196-202.
9. Clark P, Bowling A. Observational study of quality of life in NHS nursing homes and a long-stay ward for the elderly. Ageing and Society 1989; 9:123-148.
10. Carr AJ, Gibson B, Robinson PG. Measuring quality of life: Is quality of life determined by expectations or experience? BMJ 2001; 322(7296):1240-1243.
11. Ferrans CE. Quality of life as a criterion for allocation of life-sustaining treatment. In: Anderson G, Glesnes-Anderson V, editors. Health Care Ethics. Rockville: Aspen, 1987: 109-124.
12. Edlund M, Tancredi LR. Quality of life: an ideological critique. Perspect Biol Med 1985; 28(4):591-607.
13. Dolan P, Gudex C, Kind P, Williams A. Valuing health states: a comparison of methods. Journal of Health Economics 1996; 15(2):209-231.
14. Veenhoven R. The study of life satisfaction. In: Saris WE, Veenhoven R, Scherpenzeel AC, Bunting B, editors. A comparative study of satisfaction with life in Europe. Budapest: Eötvös University Press, 1996: 11-48.
15. Diener E, Suh E, Oishi S. Recent findings on subjective well-being. Indian Journal of Clinical Psychology 1997; 24(1):25-41.
16. Sartorius N. Cross-cultural comparisons of data about quality of life: A sample of issues. In: Aaronson N, Beckman J, editors. The quality of life of cancer patients. New York: Raven, 1989: 19-24.

17. Calman KC. Quality of life in cancer patients--an hypothesis. J Med Ethics 1984; 10(3):124-127.
18. Farsides B, Dunlop RJ. Measuring quality of life: Is there such a thing as a life not worth living? BMJ 2001; 322(7300):1481-1483.
19. Kinney MR. Quality of life research: rigor or rigor mortis. Cardiovasc Nurs 1995; 31(4):25-28.
20. Moons P. Why call it health-related quality of life when you mean perceived health status? Eur J Cardiovasc Nurs 2004; 3(4):275-277.
21. Zhan L. Quality of life: conceptual and measurement issues. J Adv Nurs 1992; 17(7):795-800.
22. Beckie TM, Hayduk LA. Measuring quality of life. Social Indicators Research 1997; 42(1):21-39.
23. Moons P, Van Deyk K, Marquet K, Raes E, De Bleser L, Budts W et al. Individual quality of life in adults with congenital heart disease: a paradigm shift. Eur Heart J 2005; 26(3):298-307.
24. Häyry M. Measuring the quality of life: why, how and what? In: Joyce CRB, O'Boyle CA, McGee H, editors. Individual quality of life: Approaches to conceptualisation and assessment. Amsterdam: Harwood academic publishers, 1999: 9-27.
25. Testa MA, Simonson DC. Assesment of quality-of-life outcomes. N Engl J Med 1996; 334(13):835-840.
26. Hickey A, O'Boyle CA, McGee H, Joyce CRB. The schedule for the evaluation of individual quality of life. In: Joyce CRB, O'Boyle CA, McGee H, editors. Individual quality of life: approaches to conceptualisation and assessment. Amsterdam: Harwood academic publishers, 1999: 119-133.
27. Hickey AM, Bury G, O'Boyle CA, Bradley F, O'Kelly FD, Shannon W. A new short form individual quality of life measure (SEIQoL-DW): application in a cohort of individuals with HIV/AIDS. BMJ 1996; 313(7048):29-33.
28. Hyland ME. A reformulation of quality of life for medical science. In: Joyce CRB, O'Boyle CA, McGee H, editors. Individual quality of life: approaches to conceptualisation and assessment. Amsterdam: Harwood academic publishers, 1999: 41-49.
29. Gill TM, Feinstein AR. A critical appraisal of the quality of quality-of-life measurements. JAMA 1994; 272(8):619-626.
30. Diener E, Emmons RA, Larsen RJ, Griffin S. The Satisfaction with Life Scale. Journal of Personality Assessment 1985; 49(1):71-75.
31. Badia X, Monserrat S, Roset M, Herdman M. Feasibility, validity and test-retest reliability of scaling methods for health states: the visual analogue scale and the time trade-off. Qual Life Res 1999; 8(4):303-310.
32. Pavot W, Diener E, Colvin CR, Sandvik E. Further validation of the Satisfaction with Life Scale: evidence for the cross-method convergence of well-being measures. J Pers Assess 1991; 57(1):149-161.
33. O'Boyle CA, McGee H, Hickey A, O'Malley K, Joyce CR. Individual quality of life in patients undergoing hip replacement. Lancet 1992; 339(8801):1088-1091.
34. Browne JP, O'Boyle CA, McGee HM, McDonald NJ, Joyce CRB. Development of a direct weighting procedure for quality of life domains. Qual Life Res 1997; 6(4):301-309.
35. Joyce CRB, Hickey A, McGee HM, O'Boyle CA. A theory-based method for the evaluation of individual quality of life: The SEIQoL. Qual Life Res 2003; 12(3):275-280.
36. Moons P, Marquet K, Budts W, De Geest S. Validity, reliability and responsiveness of the "Schedule for the Evaluation of Individual Quality of Life - Direct Weighting" (SEIQoL-DW) in congenital heart disease. Health Qual Life Outcomes 2004; 2(1):27.

Chapter 3

Quality of life of adults with congenital heart disease is better than that of healthy counterparts

Improvements in pediatric cardiology, intensive care medicine and cardiac surgery have resulted in decreased mortality and morbidity in patients with congenital heart disease. Due to the improved outcome, increasing attention is now being given to the quality of life of these patients, both in clinical practice and in research. Indeed, an increasing number of studies on quality of life in children, adolescents, and adults with congenital heart disease have been published over the past decades.

Reviewing the literature, we assessed the caliber of quality-of-life studies in congenital heart disease [1]. We concluded that many of the published studies have major conceptual and methodological drawbacks (see chapter 1). To address these issues, we have suggested that future quality-of-life studies must invest in a rigorous conceptualization, an adequate definition, and a sound measurement of quality of life [1].

Prior concept analyses along with the pitfalls that we identified indicate that quality of life should be defined and measured in terms of life satisfaction. Accordingly, we defined quality of life as the degree of overall life satisfaction that is positively or negatively influenced by individuals' perception of certain aspects of life important to them, including matters both related and unrelated to health [2]. The goals of the present study were to evaluate the quality of life and self-perceived health in adults with congenital heart disease using these new standards of quality-of-life assessments, and to directly compare the quality of life and health status of these patients with those of matched, healthy control participants.

METHODS

Subjects
As part of a comprehensive research project on quality of life in adults with congenital heart disease [2], 404 adult patients were matched with 404 healthy control persons according to age, sex, educational level, and occupational status (1:1 matching). Patients were recruited at the

outpatient clinic of the Adult Congenital Heart Disease Program of the University Hospitals of Leuven (Belgium). Patients were included in our study if they were 18 years or older, literate, Dutch-speaking, and gave verbal informed consent. They were excluded if it was their first visit to the outpatient clinic at the center, if they presented with mental retardation (observed or confirmed during the clinical interview), or if they were referred for or in follow-up after percutaneous closure of an atrial septal defect or a patent foramen ovale. An independent researcher obtained informed consent from patients and provided instructions on filling out the questionnaires. The researcher remained available to provide clarification if needed and to ensure that patients filled out the questionnaires independently, without interference from accompanying persons. The data collection procedure required 15–20 min.

Control subjects voluntarily participated in the study and were enrolled from a wide range of high schools, colleges, universities, companies, and administration organizations in our geographic region. We used two approaches to enroll qualifying control subjects. First, based on the matching criteria, potential control subjects were identified from the organization's personnel database. These persons were subsequently invited to participate. Second, the aim and procedure of the study was explained to the students of specific classes or to employees of the participating company by using the internal communication bulletin or in a 5-min information flash. Persons who were willing to participate could apply for the study. Their demographic characteristics were checked with the matching criteria. If a corresponding patient was included in the study, this control participant could participate. This resulted in a one-to-one matching.

Demographic and clinical characteristics of the study sample are detailed in **Table 1**. Primary medical diagnosis, treatment, and outcome in terms of quality of life and perceived health of the sub-sample in the present study did not differ from the overall population in the larger study [2], indicating that it was representative.

Variables and measurement
Quality of life
Two instruments were used to assess quality of life. Firstly, a linear analog scale (LAS) was employed. The LAS we used consisted of a vertically oriented, 10 cm line, graded with indicators ranging from 0 (worst imaginable quality of life) to 100 (best imaginable quality of life). Respondents were asked to rate their overall quality of life by marking whichever point on the scale that indicates how good or bad their quality of life is in their opinion. Psychometric properties of the LAS for the use in adults with congenital heart disease are described in **Table 2**, indicating that the LAS is valid, reliable and responsive for its purpose.

Table 1 Demographic and clinical characteristics of 404 adult patients with congenital heart disease and 404 matched healthy controls

Variable	Patients (n = 404)	Control persons (n = 404)
Sex		
Male	221 (54.7%)	221 (54.7%)
Female	183 (45.3%)	183 (45.3%)
Median age (years):	23	23
	(Q_1=20; Q_3=28.75)	(Q_1=20; Q_3=29.75)
	range 18-56	range 18-58
Marital status		
Unmarried (living with parents)	232 (57.7%)	213 (52.9%)
Living alone, divorced or widowed	35 (8.7%)	46 (11.4%)
Married or cohabiting	135 (33.6%)	144 (35.7%)
Primary medical diagnosis		
Ventricular Septal Defect	79 (19.6%)	
Tetralogy of Fallot	68 (16.8%)	
Coarctation of the aorta	62 (15.3%)	
Congenital stenosis of aortic valve	42 (10.4%)	
Pulmonary valve stenosis (congenital)	31 (7.7%)	
Complete transposition of great vessels	20 (5.0%)	
Mixed aortic valve disease	17 (4.2%)	
Ostium secundum atrial septal defect	17 (4.2%)	
Congenital mitral insufficiency	15 (3.7%)	
Univentricular heart	12 (3.0%)	
Double outlet right ventricle	7 (1.7%)	
Congenitally-corrected transposition of great vessels	5 (1.2%)	
Congenital insufficiency of aortic valve	4 (1.0%)	
Dilatation of the sinus of Valsalva	4 (1.0%)	
Congestive/dilated cardiomyopathy	3 (0.7%)	
Hypertrophic obstructive cardiomyopathy	3 (0.7%)	
Ebstein's anomaly	3 (0.7%)	
Partial anomalous pulmonary venous connection	2 (0.5%)	
Double aortic arch	2 (0.5%)	
Ostium primum defect	2 (0.5%)	
Atrio-ventricular septum defect	1 (0.2%)	
Restrictive cardiomyopathy	1 (0.2%)	
Hypoplastic right ventricle	1 (0.2%)	
Coronary artery anomaly (ALCAPA)	1 (0.2%)	
Cor triatriatum	1 (0.2%)	
Mitral valve stenosis	1 (0.2%)	
Treatment		
No treatment	121 (30%)	
Surgery	255 (63.1%)	
Catheter intervention	61 (15.1%)	
Medication	65 (16.1%)	
AICD/reconversion/pacemaker	26 (6.4%)	
NYHA class		
I	339 (84.3%)	
II	51 (12.7%)	
III	11 (2.7%)	
IV	1 (0.2%)	
Median frequency of follow-up at congenital cardiology outpatient clinic (n=581) (years)	2 (Q_1 = 1.0; Q_3 = 3.0) range 0.25-6	

AICD, Automatic Implantable Cardioverter Defibrillator; NYHA, New York Heart Association

Table 2 Psychometric properties of instrument in the present study

Variables and instruments	Number of items	Score	Test content	Relation with other variables	Reliability	Responsiveness
Quality of life						
LAS	1	0–100	H1: Respondents understand the purpose and procedure Confirmed: 100% of the patients did understand the wording and format of the LAS	H2: Because quality of life is defined as life satisfaction, the LAS is highly correlated with the SWLS Confirmed: ρ = 0.52; $P < 0.001$ H3: Because quality of life differs from health status, the LAS of quality of life is low to moderate correlated with the LAS of health status Confirmed: ρ=0.37; p<0.001	H4: Test-retest scores are highly correlated in patien with stable medical and psychosocial condition Confirmed: ICC = 0.65; $P < 0.001$	Floor scores: 0% Ceiling scores: 2.7%
SWLS	5	5–35	H5: Respondents understand the purpose and procedure Confirmed: 100% of the patients did understanc the wording and format of the SWLS	H6: Poor self-rated health is moderately associated with low levels of life satisfaction Confirmed: ρ = 0.36; $P < 0.001$	Cronbach's α = 0.70 H7: Test-retest scores are highly correlated in patien with stable medical and psychosocial condition Confirmed: ICC = 0.83; $P < 0.001$	Floor scores: 0% Ceiling scores: 1.2%
Health status						
LAS	1	0–100	H8: Respondents understand the purpose and procedure Confirmed: 100% of the patients did understand the wording and format of the LAS	H9: Because quality of life differs from health status, the LAS of quality of life is low to moderately correlated with the LAS of health status Confirmed: ρ = 0.37; $P < 0.001$ H10: The LAS of health status could differentiate between cyanotic and acyanotic patients Confirmed: cyanotic = 72.5; acyanotic = 80 (U = 4036; P = 0.01)	H11: Test-retest scores are highly correlated in patients with stable health Confirmed: ICC = 0.69; $P < 0.0001$	Floor score: 0% Ceiling scores: 3% H12: Patients who experience complications have a lower score at retest than at test Confirmed: test = 78; retest = 65 (Z = -2.927; P = 0.003)

LAS, linear analog scale; H, hypothesis; SWLS, Satisfaction with Life Scale; ICC, intra-class correlation.

Secondly, the Satisfaction with Life Scale (SWLS) [3] was used as an indicator of the quality of life. This scale consists of five statements referring to general life satisfaction. Responses were scored on a seven-point Likert scale, ranging from one (strongly disagree) to seven (strongly agree). An overall score was computed by summing the individual item scores, with the minimum possible score being five and the maximum score 35. This scale is also psychometrically sound to be used in congenital heart disease (**Table 2**).

Determinants of quality of life
Problems and concerns relevant to patients' quality of life were assessed using the Congenital Heart Disease–TNO-AZL Adult Quality of Life (CHD-TAAQOL) tool [4]. The CHD-TAAQOL was initially developed as a disease-specific tool for measuring health-related quality of life in adults with congenital heart defects. Recent experiences, however, indicate that this instrument assesses potential determinants of quality of life rather than quality of life itself [5]. The questionnaire consists of 77 items referring to specific problems or concerns of adults with congenital heart disease, such as physical functioning, symptoms, medication, activities of daily living, and social functioning. For each item, both the perceived frequency and the associated level of distress are scored. These two scales were transformed to an ordinal five-point rating scale, ranging from 0 (problem does not occur) to five (problem is very distressing).

Data on the reliability and validity of the CHD-TAAQOL are limited, because the tool is relatively new. In a first attempt to optimize construct validity, factor analysis was performed on data from 156 patients [4]. Three principal components (symptoms, impact of cardiac surveillance, and worries) comprising 26 items were identified. Based on this finding, the tool was reduced from 77 to 26 items by removing the items that were not attributed to one of the three factors. In a study of patients that received Mustard or Senning operations, however, we found that this scale reduction compromised content validity [5]. In the present study, we therefore used the initial 77 items, but limited the analyses to the item level, instead of calculating total scores or subscale scores.

Health status
Health status, as perceived by the patients, was also measured using a LAS. For its end-point indicators, this LAS used the phrases 'worst imaginable health state' (=0) as the low-end and the 'best imaginable health state' (=100) as the high-end. As part of the EuroQol instrument, this LAS is also known as the EQ-5DVAS or the EQ-5D thermometer. The EQ-5DVAS has been shown to have good validity, reliability and responsiveness when it is used in congenital heart disease (**Table 2**).

Statistical analysis

Descriptive statistics of continuous variables were expressed as medians and quartiles (Q1 and Q3) because these variables' sample values had a non-normal distribution. Frequencies and percentages were calculated for nominal variables. Because the SWLS and the CHD–TAAQOL were measured at the ordinal level, ridit analysis was used [6].

Group differences in quality of life, perceived health, and determinants of quality of life were expressed as standardized differences between patients and matched healthy control subjects. For each patient, the score of the corresponding control subject was subtracted from the patient's score and this was divided by the standard deviation of the control group, generating a standardized difference for that patient. Averaging this difference over all patients resulted in a mean standardized difference. A one sample t-test was used to evaluate whether the mean standardized differences significantly differed from zero. Two-tailed tests were used, and the level of significance was set at $P<0.05$.

RESULTS

Quality of life and perceived health

Adults with congenital heart disease perceived their quality of life to be rather good. For these patients, the median score on the LAS for quality of life was 80 (Q1=75; Q3=85.75) on a scale of 0 to 100. The median SWLS score was 28 (Q1=25; Q3=30) on a scale of 5 to 35. The median LAS score for subjective health status was 80 (Q1=70; Q3=87.75), indicating that patients perceived their health status to be good.

Analysis of the CHD-TAAQOL at the item level resulted in a ranking order of the patients' most important distressing problems or concerns (**Table 3**). Patients were most worried about the feeling that their body was less capable than they would wish. Most items in the top 10 list of determinants of quality of life, dealt with experiences about physical limitations and specific symptoms.

Table 3 Ten most important determinants of quality of life

Determinants of quality of life (n=404)	Ridit
Feeling that one's body is less capable than one would wish	0.628
Worrying about one's health	0.620
Feeling too fat or too thin	0.603
Being short of breath after strolling 1–5 km	0.602
Being so exhausted after a work day as to not be capable of anything	0.594
Excessive perspiration	0.583
Wanting to change external appearance	0.575
Worrying about job/future job	0.572
Not feeling strong enough	0.569
Dizziness	0.556

Comparison with healthy population

Compared to their healthy counterparts, adults with congenital heart disease had a significantly better quality of life, as measured with the LAS and the SWLS (**Figure 1**). Although the scores of patients and control subjects differed significant, differences were small as the mean standardized difference was less than 0.5 for both scales [7]. Self-perceived health status, however, did not differ between groups.

Problems and worries of adults with congenital heart disease, as measured with the CHD-TAAQOL, overlapped to a large extent with those identified by healthy control subjects. Patients reported significantly higher distress scores for 16 of 77 items, whereas control subjects perceived more distress for 20 items (**Figure 2**). Items that were more distressing for patients referred to specific symptoms, practical issues such as doctor visits, diet recommendations, and physical limitations. Patients reported significantly fewer difficulties or worries regarding school or work, physical appearance, sex, relationships, and friends than did their healthy counterparts.

Figure 1 Mean standardized differences (±95% confidence intervals) in quality of life and perceived health between adults with congenital heart disease and matched healthy control subjects.

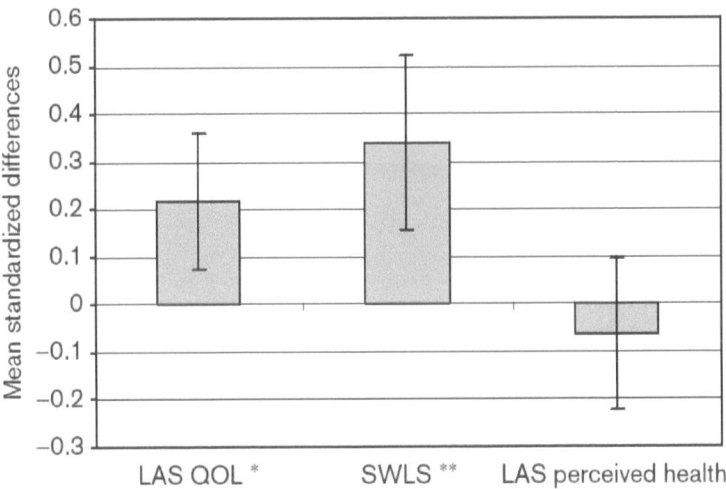

Values greater than zero indicate that the quality of life or perceived health of patients is higher than those of the control participants. Effect sizes [7] were as follows: small difference (0.2-0.5); moderate difference (0.5-0.8); large difference (≥0.8). LAS, linear analog scale; QOL, quality of life; SWLS, Satisfaction with Life Scale. *$P<0.01$; **$P<0.001$

Fig. 2 Mean standardized differences (±95% confidence intervals) in determinants of quality of life between adults with congenital heart disease and matched healthy control subjects.

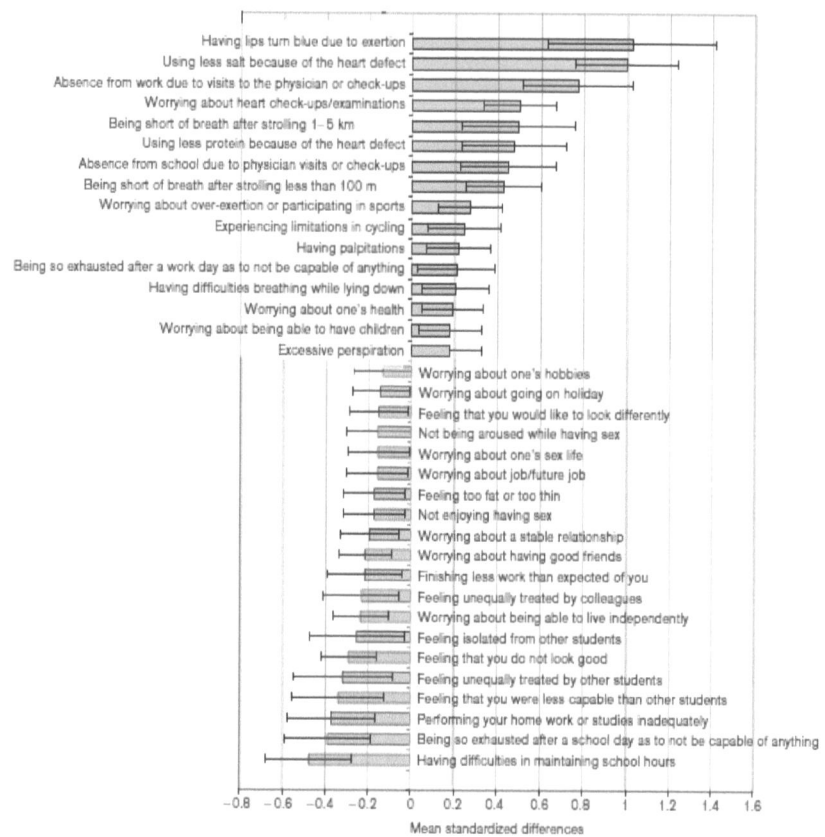

Values greater than zero indicate that patients experience more distress from that item than do the control subjects. Effect sizes [7] were as follows: small difference (0.2-0.5); moderate difference (0.5-0.8); large difference (≥0.8).

DISCUSSION

Although several studies on quality of life in adults with congenital heart disease have been published to date, it is reported that many of them are undermined to some degree by conceptual and methodological flaws [1]. Moreover, only a few studies have directly compared the quality of life in congenital heart disease patients with that in the general population. In the present study, we evaluated the quality of life and self-perceived health in adults with congenital heart disease using a design and instruments based on a sound conceptual basis. Most importantly, we directly compared the patients with matched, healthy control subjects.

We found that the quality of life in patients with congenital heart disease is perceived to be good, even better than that of their healthy counterparts. Their self-perceived health was also good and did not differ from that of the control subjects. These findings may appear to be counterintuitive at first glance and be at odds with previous studies, since these on balance have indicated that quality of life in adults with congenital heart disease is equivalent to that of the general population. Only when quality of life is assessed with a functional status instrument, do patients show a lower level of functioning than control subjects [8-10]. The disparity between our findings and those from other published studies may be due to differences in quality-of-life conceptualization and measurement. We also selected the whole spectrum of heart defects, in contrast with most other studies. Furthermore, most studies have used norm data available from the general population instead of data from patient-matched control participants. Even adjusting norm data for age and sex fails to control for differences in social and economic characteristics, which hampers the comparability of patient and control groups.

There are three potential pathways to explain the better reported quality of life in our patients with heart defects. The first possible explanation is the disability paradox [11]. Research indicated that individuals with disabilities may perceive a high quality of life if they acknowledge their impairment; if they preserve control over their body, mind, and lives; if they remain able to perform expected roles; and if they feel satisfied when comparing their self and capabilities with the conditions of others in similar situations. Conversely, factors contributing to a poor quality of life were having pain; experiencing frequent or continued fatigue; and losing control over one's body functions [11]. The characteristics of living with congenital heart disease mirror both the presence of factors contributing to an excellent quality of life and the absence of factors contributing to a poor quality of life [2].

The second pathway to explain our findings is sense of coherence [12,13] (see chapter 7). Sense of coherence is basically a measure of an individual's world view, which is enhanced by a feeling of high comprehensibility, manageability, and meaningfulness. It is hypothesized that growing up with congenital heart disease and its consequences may have positively influenced the development of sense of coherence, because patients have learnt to cope with their disease (manageability) and having had a heart operation often has a high existential meaning (meaningfulness). Because sense of coherence is strongly, positively associated with life satisfaction and quality of life [2], this may explain the better quality of life in our patients.

A final explanation for the better results in the patient group is the response shift [14]. Response shift is the change in the meaning of one's self-evaluation of a target construct as a result of a change in internal standards and values, or a redefinition of the target construct [15]. Although response shift is most pertinent in longitudinal studies, it may also affect the results of cross-sectional studies, because an interpersonal difference of internal values and standards, or interpretation of the concept may occur. It is possible that patients who grew up with congenital heart disease have developed internal values that are substantially different from those of healthy persons. More details on these three potential pathways are described elsewhere [2].

When we compared specific problems and worries of patients with those of control subjects, only 16 of 77 items were significantly more distressing for the patients. Not surprisingly, these items reflected practical issues such as doctor visits and check-ups, specific health behaviors, selected symptoms, and problems associated with physical limitations. Hence, these issues should be addressed in comprehensive healthcare programs that aim to improve patients' quality of life. Issues related to work and school, social integration, physical appearance, and sexual activities were more distressing for control subjects. This finding may be surprising, since job opportunities and social integration have been documented to be problematic in the population of patients with congenital heart disease [16-19]. Our present findings indicate, however, that, despite the risk for reduced job participation and potential suboptimal academic achievements, the patients experience fewer difficulties and worries in performing work-related and school-related activities than do their healthy counterparts.

The finding that patients perceive their health as good as control subjects, but are more worried about their health may seem contradictory. The subjective appraisal of one's own health status, however, can be considered as a cognitive process, whereas the 'health worries' from the CHD-TAAQOL is rather an emotional process since respondents are asked to rate how distressing the item is to them.

Since we have included the broad spectrum of congenital cardiac anomalies in this study, it could be questioned whether quality of life differs according to the severity of the heart defect. We found that the severity of congenital heart disease is marginally associated with patients' quality of life. This issue has been described in detail in a related paper [20] (see chapter 5).

Methodological issues

To avoid high attrition, which would consequently introduce possible selection bias, we recruited respondents at the outpatient clinic of the Adult Congenital Heart Disease Program. This resulted in a high response rate and ensured that the questionnaires were independently completed by the patient. Yet, one disadvantage of this approach is that the sample may not necessarily represent the entire population of patients with cardiac anomalies. Indeed, many patients born with heart defects are treated in the first years of life and do not need regular follow-up care at a tertiary care center. Hence, our results may only be generalized to the population of adults with congenital heart disease who are still in need of medical follow-up.

Another limitation of this study is that it was conducted at a single center. This may also compromise generalizability towards the larger population of patients with congenital heart disease.

In this study, we debarred patients with significant developmental delays from participation. We acknowledge that inclusion of this group of patients would be utmost relevant, because they may be considered as the most severely handicapped. They were excluded, however, because filling out the questionnaires used in this investigation requires intact intellectual abilities [5].

The CHD-TAAQOL was developed to be a disease-specific tool to evaluate health-related quality of life in adults with congenital heart disease [4]. In a first attempt to optimize the validity of this instrument, its scale was reduced from 77 items to 26, on the basis of factor analysis [4]. Because we previously found that this scale reduction compromised content validity [5], we used the initial 77 items in the present study. Despite the instrument's aim to assess disease-specific, health-related quality of life, we found that only 16 items of the tool were significantly more distressing for patients, whereas 20 items were more distressing for control subjects. The findings of this study therefore suggest that further validation research is needed with respect to the CHD-TAAQOL.

CONCLUSION

This study directly compared the quality of life and self-perceived health in adults with congenital heart disease with that in matched, healthy control subjects. We found that patients perceived their quality of life to be better than did their healthy counterparts, but differences were small. On the other hand, patients and healthy control subjects perceived their health status to be equivalent. Fewer issues evoked more distress in the patient group compared with the matched control persons. This finding refutes the presumed lower quality of life in patients with cardiac anomalies.

REFERENCES

1. Moons P, Van Deyk K, Budts W, De Geest S. Caliber of quality-of-life assessments in congenital heart disease: a plea for more conceptual and methodological rigor. Arch Pediatr Adolesc Med 2004; 158:1062-1069.
2. Moons P. Quality of life in adults with congenital heart disease: Beyond the quantity of life. Leuven: P. Moons; 2004.
3. Diener E, Emmons RA, Larsen RJ, Griffin S. The satisfaction with life scale. J Pers Assess 1985; 49:71-75.
4. Kamphuis M, Zwinderman KH, Vogels T, Vliegen HW, Kamphuis RP, Ottenkamp J, et al. A cardiac-specific health-related quality of life module for young adults with congenital heart disease: Development and validation. Qual Life Res 2004; 13:735-745.
5. Moons P, De Bleser L, Budts W, Sluysmans T, De Wolf D, Massin M, et al. Health status, functional abilities and quality of life following the Mustard or Senning operation. Ann Thorac Surg 2004; 77:1359-1365.
6. Sermeus W, Delesie L. Ridit analysis on ordinal data. West J Nurs Res 1996; 18:351-359.
7. Cohen J. Statistical power analysis for the behavioral sciences. Hillsdale: Lawrence Erlbaum; 1988.
8. Kamphuis M, Ottenkamp J, Vliegen HW, Vogels T, Zwinderman KH, Kamphuis RP, Verloove-Vanhorick SP. Health related quality of life and health status in adult survivors with previously operated complex congenital heart disease. Heart 2002; 87:356-362.
9. Lane DA, Lip GY, Millane TA. Quality of life in adults with congenital heart disease. Heart 2002; 88:71-75.
10. Simko LC, McGinnis KA. Quality of life experienced by adults with congenital heart disease. AACN Clin Issues 2003; 14:42-53.
11. Albrecht GL, Devlieger PJ. The disability paradox: High quality of life against all odds. Soc Sci Med 1999; 48:977-988.
12. Antonovsky A. Unraveling the mystery of health: How people manage stress and stay well. San Francisco: Jossey-Bass; 1987.
13. Moons P, Norekval TM. Is sense of coherence a pathway for improving the quality of life of patients who grow up with chronic diseases? A hypothesis. Eur J Cardiovasc Nurs 2005; 5:16-20.
14. Rapkin BD, Schwartz CE. Toward a theoretical model of quality-of-life appraisal: Implications of findings from studies of response shift. Health Qual Life Outcomes 2004; 2:14.
15. Sprangers MA, Schwartz CE. Integrating response shift into health-related quality of life research: a theoretical model. Soc Sci Med 1999; 48: 1507-1515.
16. McGrath KA, Truesdell SC. Employability and career counseling for adolescents and adults with congenital heart disease. Nurs Clin North Am 1994; 29:319-330.
17. Hart EM, Garson A. Psychosocial concerns of adults with congenital heart disease. Employability and insurability. Cardiol Clin 1993; 11:711-715.
18. Kamphuis M, Vogels T, Ottenkamp J, Van Der Wall EE, Verloove-Vanhorick SP, Vliegen HW. Employment in adults with congenital heart disease. Arch Pediatr Adolesc Med 2002; 156:1143-1148.
19. Kokkonen J, Paavilainen T. Social adaptation of young adults with congenital heart disease. Int J Cardiol 1992; 36:23-29.
20. Moons P, Van Deyk K, DeGeest S, Gewillig M, Budts W. Is the severity of congenital heart disease associated with the quality of life and perceived health of adult patients? Heart 2005; 91:1193-1198.

Chapter 4

Individual quality of life in adults with congenital heart disease: What is important for their quality of life?

The life expectancy of patients with congenital heart disease has increased substantially over the past decades. This decrease in mortality has elicited heightened interest in quality of life issues pertaining to patients with congenital heart disease. In addition to ongoing medical problems, many of these patients continually face specific psychosocial, educational, and behavioral challenges and concerns.[1] Indeed, for many of these patients, their heart defect impacts their quality of life on a daily basis.

There are two major approaches to measuring quality of life: the 'need approach' and the 'want approach'.[2] (see chapter 2) The need approach is a mainstay of quality of life studies. According to this approach, quality of life depends on fulfillment of basic needs, such as good health, sufficient mobility, good physical performance, adequate nutrition, and favorable shelter. In this approach, quality of life is measured using standardized and pre-defined questionnaires about components or determinants of quality of life. The relative importance of each of these components is assumed to be equal for all respondents. Three types of measurement are often used in this respect: (i) generic instruments, which comprehensively assess quality of life in a variety of populations; (ii) disease-specific instruments, which are developed for a particular disease or health condition; and (iii) test batteries, which employ both generic and disease-specific instruments.[3]

The want approach assumes that quality of life can only be affected by factors important to an individual.[2] For example, according to the want approach, quality of life depends on lifestyle, previous experiences, ambitions, and dreams.[2] Hence, in this approach, quality of life must be measured with instruments that permit respondents to indicate and respectively rate domains that are specifically important for their quality of life (i.e. individual quality of life). During the last decade, a paradigm shift has taken place in the measurement of quality of life, from one based on the need approach to one based on the want approach. Some now argue that the want approach is the most valid way of measuring quality of life, because it explicitly includes domains that are relevant for the respondents.[4,5] This is obviously a limitation of the need approach.

Several methods have been developed for assessing quality of life that use the want approach.[6,7] One such method is the Schedule for the Evaluation of Individual Quality of Life (SEIQoL).[6] It was developed to examine quality of life from an individual's perspective by assessing issues defined by the respondent that they feel are most important for quality of life. In contrast to pre-defined questionnaires, which assess quality of life in a more functional manner, SEIQoL reflects a more holistic view, because it considers the effects of non-disease-related aspects of life.[8] The SEIQoL, therefore, provides critical information on a patient's perspective of quality of life issues. This is important for adequate patient management in integrated healthcare programs.

Adults with congenital heart disease constitute a relatively new and growing patient population. To meet the specific needs of these patients, understanding psychosocial issues, including quality of life, is critical for developing comprehensive healthcare programs for this group of patients. Therefore, the goal of the present study was to identify specific issues, or domains, that most importantly affect the quality of life in adults with congenital heart disease. This was achieved in part by comparing differences in individual quality of life as defined by our study group with those defined by healthy counterparts.

METHODS

Study population
The present study was part of a larger research program examining the quality of life in adults with congenital heart disease, conducted from 28 November 2000 to 27 November 2002 at the University Hospitals of Leuven in Belgium.[9] In this 2 year period, 1535 outpatient visits by 1135 patients were performed. To be included in our study, the patients must have been diagnosed with congenital heart disease, were 18 years or older, literate, and Dutch-speaking. Patients meeting the following criteria were excluded: first-time patients of our outpatient clinic, mentally retarded patients (observed or confirmed during the clinical interview), referral or follow-up patients who had undergone percutaneous closure of an atrial septal defect or a patent foramen ovale because of cryptogenic stroke, or sensory or physical limitations to participate (**Figure 1**). Since this study used self-report questionnaires, eligible patients must have been able to read and write Dutch. Hence, quality of life of patients with mental retardation or illiterate patients were not addressed in this study, because these populations require a specific methodological approach, different from the methods used in this investigation.

Figure 1: Flow chart of patient selection

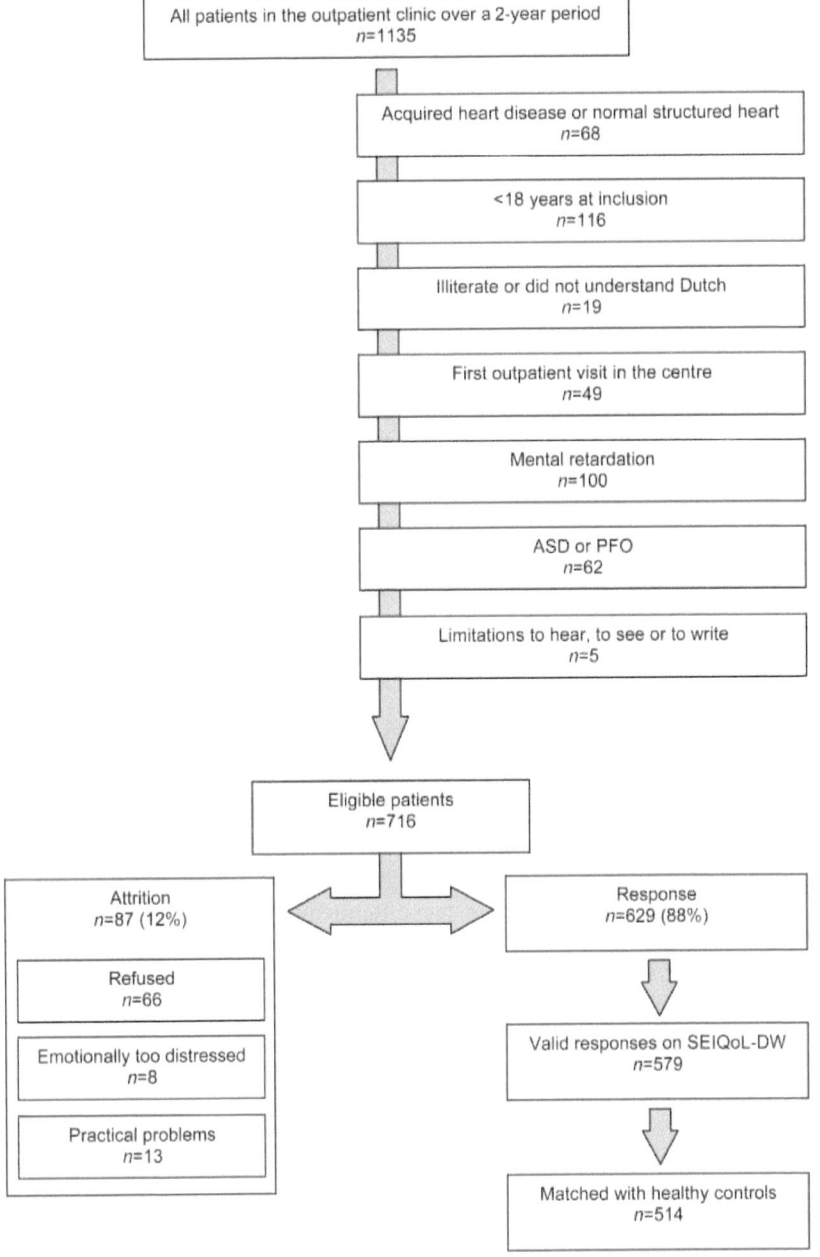

A total of 716 patients met the inclusion criteria and were asked to participate in this cross-sectional, comparative study. Of these patients, 66 subjects (9.2%) declined to participate, eight (1.1%) did not participate because they felt too emotionally distressed after the visit with the cardiologist, and 13 (1.8%) were excluded for practical reasons, resulting in a sample of 629 individuals (**Figure 1**). Since the reason not to take part in the study could very well be related to the patient's quality of life, the introduction of a potential selection bias cannot be excluded. Fifty patients did not provide valid answers, and were therefore excluded from the analysis (see Results).

To explore differences between individuals with and those without heart defects, a subsample of 514 adult patients with congenital heart disease were matched with 446 healthy control subjects according to age, gender, educational level, and occupational status (m:n matching). Control subjects were volunteers recruited from a range of high schools, colleges, universities, companies, and administration organizations in our geographical region. From the remaining 65 patients, 15 and eight patients were not selected for matching because they were disabled or received special education, respectively. For patients who were retired (n=5), or unemployed/housewife (n=30) no matching control persons could be recruited because we could not find an organization that was willing to participate. For seven patients, no control person complying with the matching criteria was available.

Variables and measurement
On the basis of a thorough conceptual foundation, we defined quality of life 'as the degree of overall life satisfaction that is positively or negatively influenced by individuals' perception of certain aspects of life important to them, including matters both related and unrelated to health'.[10] With this definition, quality of life ought to be measured in terms of life satisfaction. The SEIQoL Direct Weighting (SEIQoL-DW)[11] was used to evaluate the aspects of life that were important for individual quality of life in our subjects (i.e. determinants of quality of life). Administration of the SEIQoL-DW includes three successive stages, comprising both qualitative and quantitative assessments:

(i) Using a semi-structured interview, we asked respondents to think about their lives and designate five domains of life that they perceived as most important for their quality of life. For each domain identified, patients were also asked to elaborate more precisely about that domain, or what in particular made that domain so important to them. This elaboration allowed the investigators to gain insight into the meaning of the identified domains.

(ii) Respondents were asked to rate the actual status or level of fulfillment for each specified domain by drawing a vertical box between the terms 'worst possible' (0) and 'best possible' (100). The horizontal placement of the box corresponded to the actual status or degree of fulfillment (e.g. a box drawn toward the 100 marker indicated the highest degree of fulfillment).

(iii) Finally, respondents were asked to quantify the relative importance of each domain using a colored five-segment disc. Respondents could enlarge or reduce each segment according to their perceived relative contribution of each domain. The relative importance was expressed as a percentage.

The SEIQoL-DW permits the calculation of a single index of quality of life by summing the products of the rated level and weighting for each of the five domains. This index ranges from 0 to 100, with higher scores corresponding to higher levels of quality of life.

Although the SEIQoL-DW is known to have high face and content validity,[4,5,7,11,12] little evidence was available on other psychometric properties.[8] Using the new standards of psychometric testing, our data analyses provided additional validity evidence on test content, internal structure, and relations to other variables, as well as on the stability of the instrument.[10] Although the SEIQoL-DW cannot be considered as a measure of quality of life itself, it is a valid and reliable instrument to explore determinants for patients' quality of life.[10] Responsiveness of the SEIQoL-DW in patients with congenital heart disease might be problematic,[10] and should therefore be scrutinized in further research.

Procedure
Patients were recruited following a scheduled outpatient visit to the Adult Congenital Heart Disease Clinic. After consulting with the advanced clinical nurse practitioner and a cardiologist specialized in congenital heart defects, an independent researcher obtained informed consent from qualifying patients and provided instructions on completing the questionnaires. The researcher remained available to offer clarification if needed. Administration of the SEIQoL-DW averaged 7 min (range 3–15 min). The study protocol was approved by the local ethics committee.

Two approaches to recruit eligible control subjects were used. First, based on the matching criteria, potential control subjects were identified from the organization's personnel database. These persons were subsequently invited to participate. Second, the aim and procedure of the study was explained to the students of specific classes or to employees of the participating company by using the internal communication bulletin.

Persons who were willing to participate could apply for the study. Their demographic characteristics were checked with the matching criteria. If a corresponding patient was included in the study, this control subject could participate.

Data analysis
Both qualitative and quantitative analyses were performed. Analyses were similar to content analysis techniques. For the five patient-designated domains, a standard qualitative analytical procedure was used. The domains, as well as the reasons for why they were important, were transcribed verbatim. The individual statements, in their original form, were subsequently sorted and clustered, according to common content. Each cluster was subjectively labeled according to the best description of the meaning of the statements in that cluster. For each labeled cluster, we calculated the percentage of patients mentioning the corresponding domain. To increase objectivity in the interpretation and to monitor the clustering process, peer debriefings were organized with experts in the field of quality of life and qualitative analyses. Three independent meetings with experts were arranged to reach consensus on the labeling of clusters.

Descriptive statistics of demographic and clinical variables were expressed in percentages, medians, and quartiles. Because an m:n matching was employed, conditional logistic regression on 65 strata was used if the response variable was dichotomous. Although conditional linear mixed models have been developed to be used when response variables are continuous,[13] our data did not fulfill the normality assumptions inherent to these statistics. Therefore, we calculated a mean score per group for each stratum and compared these scores between the two groups using a Wilcoxon signed-rank test. No appropriate statistics are available for the analysis of nominal level data when samples are related but unbalanced. Therefore, we used the Chi^2 and Mann–Whitney U tests to compare some demographic and social characteristics.

All tests were two-sided. The Bonferroni correction was applied to adjust for the inflating type I error in multiple testing. For each test, 12 comparisons were made (12 domains). Therefore, the level of significance was set at $P \leq 0.004$ (0.05 divided by 12).

Since determinants of quality of life may evolve when growing older, we assessed the evolution of important quality of life domains per decade of life. For this purpose, we used the Cochran–Armitage test for trends.

Results

Patient characteristics

Of the 629 patients who were initially chosen to participate in this study, 50 were excluded because their responses were considered invalid for the following reasons: the respondents failed to completely understand the SEIQoL-DW, their answers were inaccurate, or the person accompanying the respondent interfered with the SEIQoL-DW procedure. Hence, valid data were available for 579 patients (92%), 59.9% of which were male and 40.1% were female (**Table 1**). The median age of these patients was 23 years. Given this relatively young age, the majority were unmarried and lived with their parents. Most patients were employed. Primary diagnoses exhibited most often within this sample of patients were tetralogy of Fallot, ventricular septal defect, coarctation of the aorta, aortic valve stenosis, pulmonary valve stenosis, and transposition of the great arteries (**Table 2**).

Table 1 Demographic and clinical characteristics of subjects with congenital heart disease

	n (%)
Gender (n=579)	
Male	347 (59.9%)
Female	232 (40.1%)
Median age (years)	23 (Q_1=20; Q_3=29)
	range: 18 - 66
Marital status (n=576)	
Unmarried (living with parents)	322 (55.9%)
Living alone, divorced or widowed	56 (9.7%)
Married or cohabiting	198 (34.4%)
Employment status (n=579)	
Student	167 (28.8%)
Employed	342 (59.1%)
Unemployed/Looking for work	19 (3.3%)
Unable to work/Disability	15 (2.6%)
Other	36 (6.2%)
Median frequency of follow-up at Congenital Cardiology Outpatient Clinic (years)	1.5 (Q_1=1.0; Q_3=3.0) range: 0.25 - 6

Demographic and social characteristics of the 514 patients matched with the 446 healthy control persons are compared (**Table 3**). For gender, age, employment status, the presence of children, the number of children, child wish, and the possession of a driver's license, both groups were comparable [level of significance P≤0.0055 (0.05 divided by 9)]. However, significant differences were found for educational level and marital status.

Table 2   Prevalence of primary medical diagnosis in subjects with congenital heart disease

Primary Medical Diagnosis (n = 579)	Prevalence
Tetralogy of Fallot	105 (18.1%)
Ventricular Septal Defect (VSD)	99 (17.1%)
Coarctation of the aorta	83 (14.3%)
Congenital stenosis of aortic valve	58 (10.0%)
Pulmonary valve stenosis (congenital)	41 (7.1%)
Transposition of great arteries (ventriculo-arterial discordance)	32 (5.5%)
Combined aortic valve stenosis and aortic insufficiency	26 (4.5%)
Ostium secundum atrial septal defect (ASD II)	22 (3.8%)
Congenital mitral insufficiency	20 (3.5%)
Univentricular heart	18 (3.1%)
Double outlet right ventricle	10 (1.7%)
Ebstein's anomaly	9 (1.6%)
Congenitally-corrected transposition of great vessels (double discordance)	8 (1.4%)
Congenital insufficiency of aortic valve	8 (1.4%)
Partial atrio-ventricular septum defect (ASD I)	8 (1.4%)
Congestive cardiomyopathy/ Dilated cardiomyopathy	6 (1.0%)
Dilatation of the sinus of Valsalva	4 (0.7%)
Hypertrophic obstructive cardiomyopathy	4 (0.7%)
Complete atrio-ventricular septum defect	3 (0.5%)
Restrictive cardiomyopathy	2 (0.3%)
Partial anomalous pulmonary venous connection	2 (0.3%)
Interrupted aortic arch	2 (0.3%)
Double aortic arch	2 (0.3%)
Hypoplastic right ventricle	2 (0.3%)
Coronary artery anomaly (ALCAPA)	1 (0.2%)
Patent ductus arteriosus	1 (0.2%)
Total anomalous pulmonary venous connection	1 (0.2%)
Cor triatriatum	1 (0.2%)
Mitral valve stenosis	1 (0.2%)

Individual quality of life

The SEIQoL-DW identified 12 domains that affected patient quality of life (**Table 4**). Family was the most important determinant of quality of life in adults with congenital heart disease. Job/education, friends, health, and leisure time were important determinants for 48–70% of the patients. Domains such as future, pets, environment, and nourishment were important for less than 10% of the patients sampled.

Although some domains were important for only a few patients, the actual status or level of fulfillment of all domains was rated highly (median=75), except for future. Please note that, responding to the actual status of the domain future, respondents refer to the likelihood that this domain will be fulfilled. We observed individual variability in the actual status of some domains, as illustrated by the large interquartile range of the domains future (=42) and environment (=37).

Table 3 Comparison of demographic and social characteristics of patients and healthy control subjects

	Patients (n = 514)	Controls (n=446)	p-value
Gender			1.0 *
Male	319 (62.1%)	240 (53.8%)	
Female	195 (37.9%)	206 (46.2%)	
Median age (years)	23 (Q_1=20; Q_3=28)	24 (Q_1=20; Q_3=31)	0.017 §
Educational level			0.003 †
Vocational high school	169 (32.9%)	101 (22.7%)	
Technical high school	64 (12.5%)	75 (16.9%)	
High school	45 (8.8%)	35 (7.9%)	
College	164 (32.0%)	174 (39.2%)	
University	71 (13.8%)	59 (13.3%)	
Employment status			0.959 *
Student	165 (32.1%)	157 (35.2%)	
Employed	349 (67.9%)	289 (64.8%)	
Marital status			0.005 †
Unmarried (living with parents)	300 (58.7%)	215 (48.3%)	
Living alone, divorced or widowed	48 (9.4)	55 (12.4%)	
Married or cohabiting	163 (31.9%)	175 (39.3%)	
Children			0.089 *
No	442 (86.2%)	334 (75.2%)	
Yes	71 (13.8%)	110 (24.8%)	
If yes, median number of children	2 (Q_1=1; Q_3=2)	2 (Q_1=1; Q_3=2)	0.448 §
Do you wish (more) children?			0.042 †
No	93 (18.3%)	91 (21.3%)	
Yes	295 (58.1%)	263 (61.6%)	
Don't know	120 (23.6%)	73 (17.1%)	
Driving license			0.922 †
No	113 (22.2%)	100 (22.4%)	
Yes	397 (77.8%)	346 (77.6%)	

* Conditional logistic regression; † Chi²; § Mann Whitney U test;

Table 4 Important quality of life domains reported by subjects with congenital heart disease

	Percentage of Patients Choosing Domain (n = 579)	Median Actual Status (Q1 – Q3)	Relative Importance (Q1 – Q3)
Family	464 (80.1%)	87 (75 – 94)	25% (21 – 30)
Job/education	403 (69.6%)	75 (60 – 87)	16% (12 – 22)
Friends	346 (59.8%)	82 (71 – 91)	21% (16 – 25)
Health	347 (59.1%)	79 (65 – 90)	22% (17 – 28)
Leisure time	279 (48.2%)	77 (60 – 88)	16% (12 – 20)
Personal characteristics and self-fulfillment	170 (29.4%)	78 (64 – 89)	18% (15 – 24)
Financial means and material well-being	139 (24.0%)	77 (60 – 88)	13% (10 – 19)
Important values	59 (10.2%)	77 (58 – 86)	18% (11 – 24)
Future	57 (9.8%)	69 (50 – 92)	20% (12 – 27)
Pets	44 (7.6%)	92 (76 – 99)	17% (14 – 24)
Environment	32 (5.5%)	80 (51 – 89)	15% (11 – 20)
Nourishment	23 (4.0%)	93 (69 – 99)	11% (8 – 18)

Regarding the relative importance of the respective domains, family proved to be the most significant determinant of quality of life in adults with congenital heart disease, followed by health, friends, and future (≥20%). Environment, financial means and material well-being, and nourishment were less important.

On the 0–100 scale, the overall SEIQoL-DW index score for this sample of patients was 79 (Q1=70; Q3=87), suggesting that adult patients with congenital heart disease have a relatively good quality of life.

Important quality of life domains per decade of life
We found significant differences among the respective decades of life for three domains: health, family and friends (**Figure 2**). These data show that health and family become more important with increasing age. On the other hand, friends are less frequently reported by older patients as an important quality of life domain. The observed differences in the actual status and relative importance were not statistically significant.

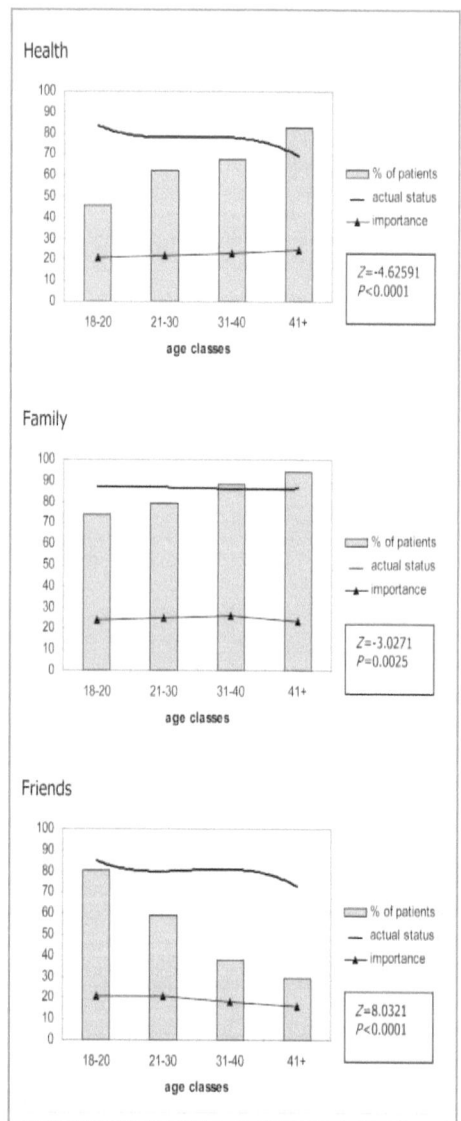

Figure 2: Important quality of life domains per decade of life

Comparison with healthy controls

Few significant differences were found in domains important for the quality of life in adults with congenital heart disease and those identified control subjects considered the domains financial means and material well-being, and future to be important determinants of quality of life. Although a few control subjects considered the domains being bereaved/loss of significant others, mental capabilities, and physical appearance/personal hygiene to be important indicators of quality of life, interestingly, patients did not consider these domains to be important for their quality of life. In addition to the lower proportion of patients indicating financial means and material well-being to be important for their quality of life, the relative importance of these domains was also significantly lower in patients than in control subjects. For the domain future, the relative importance was equal for both groups (**Table 5**).

	Number (%) of patients choosing domain			Median actual status			Relative importance (%)		
	Patients (n=514)	Controls (n=446)	p-value*	Patients (n=514)	Controls (n=446)	p-value§	Patients (n=514)	Controls (n=446)	p-value§
Family	406 (79.0)	352 (79.1)	0.882	86	82	0.091	25	24	0.006
Job/education	377 (73.3)	279 (62.7)	0.031	76	75	0.470	16	17	0.186
Friends	318 (61.9)	227 (51.0)	0.159	82	80	0.966	21	22	0.291
Health	302 (58.8)	240 (53.9)	0.161	80	83	0.038	22	25	0.014
Leisure time	250 (48.6)	172 (38.7)	0.101	77	73	0.916	16	17	0.230
Personal characteristics and self-fulfillment	156 (30.4)	135 (30.3)	0.823	79	72	0.394	18	17	0.258
Financial means and material well-being	**121 (23.5)**	**221 (49.7)**	**<0.001**	79	75	0.086	**13**	**15**	**0.002**
Important values	54 (10.5)	77 (17.3)	0.014	80	61	0.279	18	16	0.171
Future	**49 (9.5)**	**74 (16.6)**	**0.003**	66	56	0.036	19	17	0.299
Pets	37 (7.2)	11 (2.5)	0.006	91	93	0.116	16	17	0.833
Environment	29 (5.6)	32 (7.2)	0.268	80	62	0.114	15	17	0.959
Nourishment	21 (4.1)	25 (5.6)	0.438	83	85	0.463	11	15	0.528
Bereaved/loss of significant others	0 (0)	6 (1.3)	NA		35	NA		10	NA
Mental capabilities	0 (0)	5 (1.1)	NA		64	NA		11	NA
Physical appearance/personal hygiene	0 (0)	5 (1.1)	NA		65	NA		9	NA

*Conditional logistic regression; § Wilcoxon Signed Rank Test; NA= not applicable

Table 5 Comparison of important domains contributing to quality of life in subjects with congenital heart disease and healthy control subjects

Relationship to type of heart defect
We examined whether the type of congenital heart defect affected the patient's designation of domains deemed to be important for their quality of life. For this analysis, only heart defects that occurred in >5% of the sample were considered, in order to have subgroups of >30 patients. Among patients with tetralogy of Fallot, ventricular septal defect, coarctation of the aorta, congenital stenosis of the aortic valve, pulmonary valve stenosis, or transposition of the great arteries, no differences were found in the percentage of patients who identified respective domains, the actual status or relative importance. This indicates that the type of heart defect does not impact individual quality of life.

DISCUSSION

Since mortality and morbidity of patients with congenital heart disease have decreased substantially in recent decades, interest has increased greatly in issues relating to quality of life in this patient population. To date, all published studies examining quality of life issues in adults with congenital heart disease have used the need approach.[14-32] In these studies, quality of life was measured from a functional or socioeconomic, rather than an individual, perspective. The former approach typically uses standardized questionnaires or classification systems. By assessing individual quality of life, on the other hand, researchers can take into account the unique perspective of individual patients. Evaluation of individual quality of life with the want approach is therefore more suitable because it circumvents problems inherent to standardized instruments (e.g. ratings based on arbitrary topics and equal weightings of questionnaires). Indeed, by using the want approach, a researcher recognizes that, in different individuals, different variables influence quality of life and that these variables do not equally affect all individuals.[4] Acknowledging the validity of this paradigm shift, we investigated issues important for quality of life in a large sample of adults with congenital heart disease.

We found 12 important domains that contribute to the quality of life of patients with congenital heart disease. The majority of patients identified general issues, such as family, job/education, friends, and health to be important determinants of quality of life. The relative importance was highest for family, then health, friends, and future. This indicates that while job/education was, for many patients, an important determinant of quality of life, it was considered less important when compared with the other nominated domains. Only a few respondents identified concerns about their future as an important indicator of quality of life, although its relative importance was higher compared with that of many other domains.

Quality of life research often focuses on health-related quality of life. Indeed, patients' health is consistently identified as an important determinant of quality of life. However, in the present study, only 59% of the patients with congenital heart disease identified health as an important determinant of quality of life. Moreover, fairly equal numbers of patients and healthy control subjects identified health as important. This confirms that, by focusing on health-related quality of life, investigators substantially overestimate the impact of health-related factors and seriously undervalue the effect of non-medical phenomena.[5]

Our findings identified only two significant differences in important determinants of quality of life between patients with congenital heart disease and healthy persons without heart defects. Financial means and material well-being was an important determinant in twice as many control subjects as patients. The relative importance of this domain was also higher in controls than in patients. Severe heart conditions or previous operations prompt patients to put material aspects in proper perspective. This could potentially explain why fewer patients consider financial means and material well-being to be important.

The present study also revealed that the type of heart defect does not impact factors deemed important for quality of life in adults with congenital heart disease, neither the actual status nor relative importance of the respective domains. This is in line with the finding that the quality of life in our patient sample was only marginally associated with the severity of the heart defect.[33] It can therefore be assumed that patients with severe conditions do not necessarily consider other aspects of life as significant.

Implications
This investigation provides crucial information for healthcare professionals to understand better the consequences of heart defects on patients' quality of life. This study goes beyond the traditional focus of functionality problems by providing a holistic outlook on living with congenital heart disease. This holistic approach is key in comprehensive, interdisciplinary healthcare programs for these patients.

The employment of the SEIQoL-DW in this study supports the utility of this instrument to practitioners interested in measuring their patients' quality of life for clinical purposes. The time needed for completing the SEIQoL-DW is acceptable (average 7 min), and analysis—which is complex if used in research—is not necessary because only the individual responses are relevant.

Methodological issues

This article reports the application of a relatively new method of measuring quality of life in a sample of adults with congenital heart disease. The use of a patient-centered, individualized measure, such as the SEIQoL-DW, is more appropriate than standardized instruments,[34] because it provides a detailed picture of quality of life issues relevant to patients. Moreover, the SEIQoL-DW counters common problems inherent to most quality of life measures (e.g. focusing primarily on limitations and impediments, without considering positive elements that contribute favorably to quality of life). Indeed, quality of life is increasingly considered to be a positivistic concept.[10]

Despite these positive aspects, there are specific problems with individualized measures of quality of life. Some patients may have difficulty understanding the system.[8,34] In the present study, this problem was observed in 8% or 50 of the 629 patients. These patients were excluded from the analysis without affecting the sample size. Furthermore, the interpretation and analysis of data stemming from individualized measures is complex,[34] mainly because the data are qualitative. To address this issue, we used a qualitative analysis procedure that is similar to content analysis techniques. To mitigate subjectivity in the interpretation of data, final labeling was done in consensus meetings with experts in quality of life and qualitative research. Although the data collection and analysis may be complex, we have demonstrated that it is feasible to use the SEIQoL-DW in large samples. Indeed, this is the first large-scale study using an individualized quality of life instrument.

This study favorably used a large sample size. Since we enrolled patients from an outpatient clinic of a tertiary care centre, it may be argued that the sample was not representative of the entire population of adults with congenital heart disease. Many patients who are born with a rather benign cardiac anomaly are treated in the first years of life and do not need continuing check-ups at a university hospital. In addition, the strict inclusion and exclusion criteria implied that the sample was not even, as such, representative of all patients attending the outpatient clinic. We did not include patients under 18 years of age, and patients with mental retardation. The former group was excluded because questionnaires developed for adult populations are not valid to be used in adolescents. The latter group was debarred from inclusion because self-report by questionnaires requires intact intellectual abilities.

Twelve per cent of the eligible patients did not participate in the study. Since the reason not to take part in the study could very well be related to the patient's quality of life, the introduction of a potential selection bias—although limited—could not be excluded. A possible under-representation of specific heart defects in our patient sample, however, failed to affect our results since we showed that both quality of life[33] and its determinants (present study) are not influenced by the type of heart defect exhibited by the patients studied.

Although this study meets the new emerging standards of quality of life measurement, it does not fully dismiss the utility of generic and disease-specific instruments in measuring specific components of quality of life. While these instruments may not measure all aspects of quality of life, they may be useful in measuring disability related to specific diseases and effectiveness of treatment. Hence, such instruments may identify actionable items with respect to self-perceived health status of functional abilities.

CONCLUSION

During the past decade, a paradigm shift has occurred in the measurement of quality of life, from one based on the need approach to one based on the want approach. Individual quality of life assessment in adults with congenital heart disease provides a detailed picture of issues relevant for patients' quality of life. Although some domains were reported by only a few patients, these had high fulfillment and relative importance for them. Comparison of quality of life measures derived from healthy control subjects with those from patients with congenital heart disease indicated that both groups basically perceive the same issues to be important. This investigation provides crucial information for healthcare professionals to understand the consequences of heart defects on patients' quality of life better. Issues that arose in this study should be addressed in comprehensive healthcare programs that aim to improve patients' quality of life.

REFERENCES

1. Moons P, De Geest S, Budts W. Comprehensive care for adults with congenital heart disease: expanding roles for nurses. Eur J Cardiovasc Nurs 2002;1:23-28.
2. Häyry M. Measuring the quality of life: why, how and what? In: Joyce CRB, O'Boyle CA, McGee H, eds. Individual Quality of Life: Approaches to Conceptualism and Assessment. Amsterdam: Harwood Academic Publishers; 1999. p9-27.
3. Testa MA, Simonson DC. Assesment of quality-of-life outcomes. N Engl J Med 1996;334:835-840.
4. Hickey AM, Bury G, O'Boyle CA et al. A new short form individual quality of life measure (SEIQoL-DW): application in a cohort of individuals with HIV/AIDS. Br Med J 1996;313:29-33.
5. Gill TM, Feinstein AR. A critical appraisal of the quality of quality-oflife measurements. JAMA 1994;272:619-626.
6. Browne JP, McGee HM, O'Boyle CA. Conceptual approaches to the assessment of quality of life. Psychol Health 1997;12:737-751.
7. Garratt AM, Ruta DA. The patient generated index. In: Joyce CRB, O'Boyle CA, McGee H, eds. Individual Quality of Life: Approaches to Conceptualism and Assessment. Amsterdam: Harwood Academic Publishers; 1999. p105-118.
8. Macduff C. Respondent-generated quality of life measures: useful tools for nursing or more fool's gold? J Adv Nurs 2000;32:375-382.

9. Moons P. *Quality of Life in Adults with Congenital Heart Disease: Beyond the Quantity of Life.* Leuven: P. Moons; 2004.
10. Moons P, Marquet K, Budts Wet al. Validity, reliability and responsiveness of the 'Schedule for the Evaluation of Individual Quality of Life— Direct Weighting' (SEIQoL-DW) in congenital heart disease. *Health Qual Life Outcomes* 2004;2:27.
11. Browne JP, O'Boyle CA, McGee HM et al. Development of a direct weighting procedure for quality of life domains. *Qual Life Res* 1997;6:301-309.
12. Hickey A, O'Boyle CA, McGee H et al. The schedule for the evaluation of individual quality of life. In: Joyce CRB, O'Boyle CA, McGee H, eds. *Individual Quality of Life: Approaches to Conceptualism and Assessment.* Amsterdam: Harwood Academic Publishers; 1999. p119-133.
13. Verbeke G, Spiessens B, Lesaffre E. Conditional linear mixed models. *Am Stat* 2001;55:25-34.
14. Aigueperse J, Marechal MC. [Evaluation of the quality of life in adulthood of 158 patients surgically-treated for tetralogy of Fallot]. *Arch Mal Coeur Vaiss* 1991;84:685-690.
15. Daliento L, Somerville J, Presbitero P et al. Eisenmenger syndrome. Factors relating to deterioration and death. *Eur Heart J* 1998;19: 1845-1855.
16. Gersony WM, Hayes CJ, Driscoll DJ et al. Second natural history study of congenital heart defects. Quality of life of patients with aortic stenosis, pulmonary stenosis, or ventricular septal defect. *Circulation* 1993;87(Suppl.):I52-I65.
17. Immer FF, Seiler AM, Stocker F. [Status and after-care of young adults with congenital heart defects]. *Schweiz Med Wochenschr* 1998;128:1012-1019.
18. Kamphuis M, Ottenkamp J, Vliegen HW et al. Health related quality of life and health status in adult survivors with previously operated complex congenital heart disease. *Heart* 2002;87:356-362.
19. Lane DA, Lip GY, Millane TA. Quality of life in adults with congenital heart disease. *Heart* 2002;88:71-75.
20. Miyamura H, Takahashi M, Sugawara M et al. The long-term influence of pulmonary valve regurgitation following repair of tetralogy of Fallot: does preservation of the pulmonary valve ring affect quality of life? *Surg Today* 1996;26:603-606.
21. Peters KF, Kong F, Hanslo M et al. Living with Marfan syndrome III. Quality of life and reproductive planning. *Clin Genet* 2002;62:110-120.
22. Pressley JC, Wharton JM, Tang ASL et al. Effect of Ebsteins-anomaly on short-term and long-term outcome of surgically treated patients with Wolff-Parkinson-White Syndrome. *Circulation* 1992;86:1147-1155.
23. Rietveld S, Mulder BJ, van Beest I et al. Negative thoughts in adults with congenital heart disease. *Int J Cardiol* 2002;86:19-26.
24. Saliba Z, Butera G, Bonnet D et al. Quality of life and perceived health status in surviving adults with univentricular heart. *Heart* 2001;86:69-73.
25. Sandoval J, Aguirre JS, Pulido T et al. Nocturnal oxygen therapy in patients with the Eisenmenger syndrome. *Am J Resp Crit Care Med* 2001;164:1682-1687.
26. Stewart AB, Ahmed R, Travill CM et al. Coarctation of the aorta life and health 20-44 years after surgical repair. *Br Heart J* 1993;69:65-70.
27. Sugimoto S, Takagi N, Hachiro Y et al. High frequency of arrhythmias after Fontan operation indicates earlier anticoagulant therapy. *Int J Cardiol* 2001;78:33-39.
28. Ternestedt BM, Wall K, Oddsson H et al. Quality of life 20 and 30 years after surgery in patients operated on for tetralogy of Fallot and for atrial septal defect. *Pediatr Cardiol* 2001;22:128-132.
29. Verbraecken J, Declerck A, Van de Heyning P et al. Evaluation for sleep apnea in patients with Ehlers-Danlos syndrome and Marfan: a questionnaire study. *Clin Genet* 2001;60:360-365.
30. Vogel M, Berger F, Kramer A et al. Diagnose und chirurgische Behandlung von Vorhofseptumdefekten im Erwachsenenalter [Diagnosis and surgical treatment of atrial septal defects in adults]. *Dtsch Med Wochenschr* 1999;124:35-38.
31. Walker WT, Temple IK, Gnanapragasam JP et al. Quality of life after repair of tetralogy of Fallot. *Cardiol Young* 2002;12:549-553.
32. Wilson NJ, Clarkson PM, Barratt-Boyes BG et al. Long-term outcome after the mustard repair for simple transposition of the great arteries. 28-year follow-up. *J Am Coll Cardiol* 1998;32:758-765.
33. Moons P, Van Deyk K, De Geest S et al. Is the severity of congenital heart disease associated with patients' quality of life and perceived health status? *Heart* 2005;91:1193-1198.
34. Carr AJ, Higginson IJ. Measuring quality of life: are quality of life measures patient centred? *Br Med J* 2001;322:1357-1360.

Chapter 5

Quality of life of adults with congenital heart disease is marginally associated with disease severity

Congenital heart diseases comprise a wide spectrum of heart defects with varying levels of severity. The type of heart defect may affect the progress of the disease, the prognosis, and patients' ability to carry out normal functions. Indeed, some conditions, such as mild valvar disease or a small ventricular septal defect, do not require specific treatment or specialized follow up.[1] Conversely, more complex defects such as a univentricular heart or transposition of the great arteries require surgical treatment and lifelong follow up care in a tertiary care centre specialized in pediatric or adult congenital heart disease.[1] In general, more severe heart defects are associated with worse outcomes.[2]

In addition to the medical problems, many patients with congenital heart disease are facing specific psychosocial, educational, and behavioral challenges and issues. In this respect, the feeling of being different from peers, social impediments due to physical restrictions, and problems obtaining employment and insurance are often reported.[3] In many patients, congenital heart disease can be considered to be a chronic condition. This is particularly so when a patient's daily life is impeded by the long term nature of congenital heart disease, when there is a prevailing uncertainty with respect to the course of the illness and its prognosis, and when the patient experiences symptoms of the illness and restrictions in the level of activity.[4] It is assumed that these barriers influence patients' quality of life.[5] It is, however, uncertain whether the quality of life is associated with the severity of the congenital heart disease.

Few studies have attempted to examine the relation between disease severity and the quality of life of adults with congenital heart disease.[6-8] A potential relation between severity and quality of life may also be inferred from a series of studies that have applied the same instrument in different populations of heart defects.[9-12] In these studies, quality of life was measured in terms of either subjective health status,[6,9-12] the emotional response to health problems,[8] or external life conditions, interpersonal relationships, and internal psychological states.[7] Patients were categorized according to the severity of their disease, based on the initial diagnosis,[7,9-12] the New York Heart Association (NYHA) functional class, the ability index of Somerville, and criteria such as cyanosis,[6] arrhythmia, cardiac failure, and residual defects.[8]

Some associations were found between functional class and aspects of subjective health status. Although most studies have defined quality of life in terms of health status, there is more evidence that quality of life and health status are conceptually different issues.[13,14] It is therefore not appropriate to use a subjective assessment of health status as a measure of quality of life. Moreover, the respective studies measured disease severity in various ways. Indeed, disease severity is a problematic concept with respect to congenital heart disease, since several issues such as initial diagnosis, the course of the illness, functional status, or prognosis may reflect the severity of the disease in each patient. A comprehensive assessment of disease severity in congenital heart defects therefore requires an evaluation of the respective aspects. An indicator of severity is not only the heart defect itself or patients' functional class but also the number of surgical and interventional procedures or the expected course duration.

The absence of a comprehensive assessment of disease severity and the various approaches to quality of life investigations make the available study results inconclusive. This study therefore focused on exploring the association between the various indicators of congenital heart disease severity and on both the quality of life and the perceived health of adult patients, based on a sound conceptual foundation.

PATIENTS AND METHODS

Study population
During a two year period, all adult (> 18 years old), literate, Dutch speaking patients who visited the outpatient clinic for congenital heart disease at the University Hospital of Leuven, Belgium, were asked to participate in the study. Patients were excluded if it was their first visit to the outpatient clinic at the center, if they were assessed as having learning disabilities during the clinical interview, or if they were referred for or in follow up after percutaneous closure of an atrial septal defect or a patent foramen ovale. Informed consent was provided orally.

Seven hundred and sixteen patients with congenital heart disease met the inclusion criteria. However, 66 (9.2%) of these patients refused to participate in the study, eight (1.1%) felt too emotionally distressed to participate because the cardiologist just told them that they needed a reoperation or that pregnancy was contraindicated, and 13 (1.8%) were not included for practical reasons (for example, further technical investigations, taxi was waiting), yielding a sample of 629 patients. **Table 1** summarizes the demographical and clinical characteristics of the study sample. Three hundred and seventy eight male (60.1%) and 251 (39.9%) female patients were included. The median age was 24 years. The most prevalent primary diagnoses were tetralogy of Fallot and ventricular septal defect. **Table 1** describes only the six most prevalent heart defects, occurring in more than 5% of the patient sample.

Table 1: Demographic and clinical characteristics of 629 adult patients with congenital heart disease

Variable	
Gender: (n=629)	
Male	378 (60.1%)
Female	251 (39.9%)
Median age (years) (n=629)	24 (Q_1=20; Q_3=29)
	range 18 – 66
Marital status: (n=626)	
Unmarried (living with parents)	346 (55.3%)
Living alone, divorced or widowed	60 (9.6%)
Married or cohabiting	220 (35.1%)
Employment status: (n=629)	
Student	175 (27.8%)
Blue collar worker	149 (23.7%)
White collar worker	189 (30.0%)
Independent	37 (5.9%)
Unemployed/Looking for work	25 (4.0%)
Home wife	12 (1.9%)
Retired	5 (0.8%)
Not able to work/disability	17 (2.7%)
Other	20 (3.2%)
Primary medical diagnosis:	
Tetralogy of Fallot	112 (17.8%)
Ventricular Septal Defect (VSD)	108 (17.2%)
Coarctation of the aorta	89 (14.1%)
Congenital stenosis of aortic valve	65 (10.3%)
Pulmonary valve stenosis (congenital)	48 (7.6%)
Complete transposition of great vessels	37 (5.9%)

Variables and measurement
Disease severity
Various components of congenital heart disease severity were measured: initial diagnosis; illness course; and current functional status (**table 2**).[1,15-18] To determine the need for specialized care, Task Force 1 of the 32nd Bethesda Conference of the American College of Cardiology categorized congenital heart diseases into three classes, mild, moderate, and severe heart defects,[1] based on the initial diagnosis or specific types of operations (**table 2**).

Table 2: Classification systems to categorize patients with congenital heart disease according to the severity of the disease

Classification systems	Prevalence
Initial diagnosis: (n=629)	
• Task Force 1 of the 32nd Bethesda conference of the American College of Cardiology [1]	
- Mild: (e.g. isolated aortic valve disease, closed ASD without residua)	164 (26.1%)
- Moderate: (e.g. coarctation of the aorta, tetralogy of Fallot)	365 (58.0%)
- Severe: (e.g. Fontan operation, Eisenmenger, double outlet ventricle)	100 (15.9%)
Illness course: (n=629)	
• Disease Severity Index [15]	
- Low: maximal 1 cardiovascular operation or 1 catheterization procedure	404 (64.2%)
- Moderate: more than 1 cardiovascular operation or catheterization	203 (32.3%)
- High: persistent cyanosis, <92% oxygen saturation at rest, or single ventricle physiology.	22 (3.5%)
Current functional status: (n=627)	
• NYHA functional class [16]:	
-Class I: Patients with cardiac disease but without resulting limitation of physical activity. Ordinary physical activity does not cause undue fatigue, palpitation, dyspnea or anginal pain.	511 (81.5%)
-Class II: Patients with cardiac disease resulting in slight limitation of physical activity. They are comfortable at rest. Ordinary physical activity results in fatigue, palpitation, dyspnea or anginal pain.	85 (13.6%)
-Class III: Patients with cardiac disease resulting in marked limitation of physical activity. They are comfortable at rest. Less than ordinary activity causes fatigue, palpitation, dyspnea or anginal pain.	26 (4.1%)
-Class IV: Patients with cardiac disease resulting in inability to carry on any physical activity without discomfort. Symptoms of heart failure or the anginal syndrome may be present even at rest. If any physical activity is undertaken, discomfort increases.	5 (0.8%)
• Ability Index [17]: (n=628)	
- Class 1: Normal life: full-time work or school, pregnancy poses no health risk	524 (83.4%)
- Class 2: Able to work: intermittent symptoms, interference with life, pregnancy possible	78 (12.4%)
- Class 3: Unable to work: limitation of all activities, pregnancy poses health risk	24 (3.8%)
- Class 4: Extreme limitation: dependent, almost house-bound	2 (0.3%)
• Congenital heart disease functional index [18] (n=628)	
- Class 1: No surgery, good clinical status, medical follow-up not strictly necessary	24 (3.8%)
- Class 2: With or without surgery, functionally perfect, postoperative normalization of clinical condition, medical check-up every 3 to 5 years, competitive sports permitted.	221 (35.2%)
- Class 3: With or without surgery, functionally good, medical restrictions, medical check-up every 1 to 2 years, recreational sports permitted.	355 (56.5%)
- Class 4: With or without surgery, moderate functional status, functioning at own pace, medical check-up every year.	23 (3.7%)
- Class 5: With or without palliative surgery, bad functional status, cyanosis, medical check-up every 6 to 12 months.	5 (0.8%)
• Left Ventricular Ejection Fraction	Median: 62 (IQR: 15)

IQR: Inter Quartile Range

With respect to health services research, the disease severity index was developed to reflect the course of the illness.[15] The disease severity index encompasses three categories. "Low severity" was reserved for patients who had undergone a maximum of one cardiovascular operation or one catheterization procedure. Patients who had undergone more than one cardiovascular operation or catheterization were placed in the "moderate severity" group. Lastly, patients with persistent cyanosis, <92% oxygen saturation at rest, or single ventricle physiology were placed in the "high severity" group (**table 2**).

To assess the current functional status, three classification methods were used: the NYHA functional class,[16] the ability index,[17] and the congenital heart disease functional index, which was developed by the department's research group for a previous study.[18] The ability index and the congenital heart disease functional class are specifically designed for adults with congenital heart disease, whereas the NYHA classification was initially developed for patients with heart failure and later on adapted for patients with angina.[16] A fourth indicator for patients' functional status was the left ventricular ejection fraction, as measured by echocardiography. This parameter is traditionally used by cardiologists as an indicator of patients' functioning.

Quality of life
Although the concept of quality of life is often discussed in the biomedical literature, there is still no consensus on its definition, conceptualization, or measurement (see chapter 2). In preparation for this study, we evaluated the different conceptualizations of quality of life. For this evaluation, we identified six critical conceptual pitfalls regarding this concept (see chapter 2). phenomena.

Relying on a critical appraisal of quality-of-life studies,[19] published concept analyses of quality of life[20-22] and considering the pitfalls described in the literature,[28] it is indicated that quality of life should be defined and measured in terms of life satisfaction. Therefore, we defined quality of life as "the degree of overall life satisfaction that is positively or negatively influenced by people's perception of certain aspects of life important to them, including matters both related and unrelated to health" (see chapter 1).

Linear analogue scale
The overall quality of life was measured with a linear analogue scale. This is a vertical, graded, 10 cm line, ranging from the "worst imaginable quality of life" (score of 0) to the "best imaginable quality of life" (score of 100). The use of this linear analogue scale allows patients to give their own rating of their overall perceived quality of life. Linear analogue scales

are widely used in quality of life research, particularly in cancer populations.[23] It can be used to measure a variety of symptoms and aspects of functioning, as well as overall quality of life.[23,24] We used the linear analogue scale in this study because of its advantages of being easy to use[25] and less burdensome for respondents.[26] This simplicity and ease of use may result in high response rates and operational efficiency of the study.[24] Despite their simplicity, such analogue scales have been shown in several studies to be valid, reliable, and responsive to changes in clinical conditions.[23,24,27] We explored some lines of evidence on validity, reliability, and responsiveness of the linear analogue scale for quality of life in adults with congenital heart disease, indicating good psychometric properties for the use in this population of patients. Details of the psychometric evidence are described elsewhere.[28]

Satisfaction with life scale
Because the quality of life was defined in terms of life satisfaction, the satisfaction with life scale[29] was used as a second indicator of quality of life. This instrument comprises five statements and seven response categories, ranging from "strongly disagree" to "strongly agree". An aggregate score can be obtained by summing the scores of the individual items. The minimum score of life satisfaction is 5 and the maximum score is 35. The validity and reliability have been extensively assessed in previous studies and indicate good psychometric properties.[30] For their use with patients with congenital heart disease, we also found this instrument to be psychometrically sound.[28] (see chapter 3)

Schedule for the evaluation of individual quality of life – direct weighting
To explore the determinants of quality of life, we used the schedule for the evaluation of individual quality of life-direct weighting (SEIQoL-DW).[31] (see chapter 4) The SEIQoL-DW was developed to examine quality of life from an individual perspective. It consists of three successive steps: firstly, the respondent nominates the five areas that are most important for his or her quality of life; secondly, the actual status of each specified area is rated from 0 to 100 on a visual analogue scale; and, thirdly, the relative importance of each selected area is quantified relative to each other area with the use of a five segment disk. The use of SEIQoL-DW overcomes the problem of predetermined questions, which assumes that each person's quality of life is influenced by the same determinants and that different aspects of life are equally important for all people.[32] We evaluated validity, reliability, and responsiveness of the SEIQoL-DW for use in adults with congenital heart disease.[33] Although the SEIQoL-DW cannot be regarded as a measure of quality of life itself, it is a valid and reliable instrument to explore determinants for patients' quality of life.[33] Responsiveness of the SEIQoL-DW in patients with congenital heart disease may be problematic.[33] The use of the SEIQoL-DW allows the

calculation of a single index by summing the products of the rated level and applying weights for each of the five areas. This index ranges from 0 to 100. Note, however, that the SEIQoL-DW index cannot be regarded as a quality of life index but rather as an aggregate score of the most important determinants.

Health status
Because there is a substantial difference between quality of life and self perceived health, we also measured health status in this study. Subjectively perceived health status was measured with a linear analogue scale ranging from the "worst imaginable health state" (score of 0) to the "best imaginable health state" (score of 100). This linear analogue scale is part of the EuroQol instrument and previous studies have reported its good validity and reliability.[34] Also in adults with congenital heart disease, this linear analogue scale has been shown to be valid, reliable, and responsive.[28]

Procedure
After the advanced practice nurse and the cardiologist saw the patients during their scheduled visit at the outpatient clinic, an independent researcher approached the patients to explain the purpose, procedure, and time required to participate in the study. Patients were instructed on how to fill out the questionnaires after giving oral informed consent. The researcher stayed with the patient to provide clarification if needed and to ensure that patients filled out the questionnaires independently, without assistance from accompanying people. The questionnaires were checked for completeness and patients were asked to complete missing data if necessary. The data collection procedure lasted about 15-20 minutes. This study was approved by the local ethics committee and has therefore been performed in accordance with international ethical standards.

One cardiologist scored the NYHA, ability index, and congenital heart disease functional index based on data from the clinical examination. Interrater reliability was therefore not an issue in this study. The cardiologist was blinded as to other outcomes. Data on left ventricular ejection fraction were retrieved from the medical record.

Statistical analysis
The data were analyzed with SPSS 9.0 (SPSS Inc, Chicago, Illinois, USA). Nominal level data were expressed in percentages. After having been checked for normality, medians and first (Q1) and third quartiles (Q3) were calculated because continuous variables were not normally distributed. Spearman's correlation coefficients were calculated to evaluate the relation between the severity of the congenital heart disease and quality of life. Cyanotic and acyanotic patients were compared by the

Mann-Whitney U test. All tests were two sided with a level of significance set at p < 0.05. The Bonferroni correction was applied to adjust for the inflating type I error in multiple testing.

Since the satisfaction with life scale is an ordinal level instrument, summation of the scores of the individual items is not appropriate.[35] Yet, in the descriptive statistics, we calculated an overall score by summing the items scores to allow comparison with published data. For the inferential statistics, however, we transformed the ordinal scale into a probability scale by means of ridit analysis.[35] A ridit was calculated for each patient, representing an aggregate score over all items for that patient.

RESULTS

Disease severity
According to the initial diagnosis based on the Task Force 1 classification, a majority of the patients were classified as having moderate congenital heart disease (**table 2**). In contrast, the disease severity index classified 64.2% as having a mild heart defect. The NYHA classification and the ability index were fairly comparable with 81.5% and 83.4% of patients, respectively, in class I. The congenital heart disease functional index placed 56.5% of the patients in class 3 (**table 2**). The median left ventricular ejection fraction was available for 491 patients. The median ejection fraction was 62%.

Frequency distributions indicate that these classification schemes measure different indicators of disease severity. This was confirmed by the correlation coefficients between the respective classifications, which ranged from 0.25–0.49, except for the relation between NYHA and ability index (r_s = 0.86).

Quality of life and perceived health
Overall, the quality of life of adults with congenital heart disease was good. The median scores on the linear analogue scale and the satisfaction with life scale were 80 (Q1=75, Q3=87) and 28 (Q1=24, Q3=30), respectively. The median SEIQoL-DW index was 79.04 (Q1=69.56, Q3=87.20). Patients perceived their health to be good, the median linear analogue scale score being 80 (Q1=70, Q3=90).

Since we defined quality of life in terms of life satisfaction, we assumed that the linear analogue scale and the satisfaction with life scale are highly interrelating. We found a correlation coefficient of 0.52 (p<0.001). According to the cut off boundaries for small (0.1–0.3), moderate (0.3–0.5), and large correlations (>0.5),[36] both scales can be regarded as highly interrelating. On the other hand, the expected low to moderate correlation with the SEIQoL-DW ($r_s=0.42$, $p<0.001$) and the linear analogue scale of health status ($r_s=0.37$, $p<0.001$) was confirmed. The correlation between the SEIQoL-DW and the linear analogue scale of health status was even lower ($r_s=0.31$, $p<0.001$).

Relation between disease severity and quality of life

Scores derived from the disease severity classification systems indicated a weak and negative association with quality of life parameters and perceived health (**table 3**). The correlations were significant only for parameters reflecting functional status, such as NYHA, ability index, and congenital heart disease functional index. The highest correlations with functional status were found for satisfaction with life and perceived health.

Table 3: Spearman's rho correlation matrix for severity of congenital heart disease versus quality of life and health status

	LAS Quality of life	SWLS	SEIQoL-DW	LAS Health status
Task Force	-0.05	-0.06	-0.08	-0.10
Disease Severity Index	-0.09	-0.09	-0.05	-0.12
Functional status				
- NYHA	-0.20*	-0.28*	-0.18*	-0.27*
- Ability Index	-0.18*	-0.25*	-0.13*	-0.24*
- Congenital Heart Disease Functional Index	-0.11	-0.07	-0.15*	-0.20*
- Left Ventricular Ejection Fraction	0.10	0.07	0.06	0.04

SWLS= Satisfaction with Life Scale; * Bonferroni correction: $p<0.0025$

Comparison of the 20 patients with cyanotic conditions versus the 609 patients with acyanotic conditions showed that there was no significant difference (Bonferroni correction: $p<0.0125$) in quality of life parameters. However, health status was perceived to be significantly lower (U=4036, p=0.01) by cyanotic patients (median=72.5, Q1=60.5, Q3=80) than by acyanotic patients (median=80, Q1=70, Q3=90).

DISCUSSION

This is the first study that comprehensively explored the association between the severity of congenital heart disease and quality of life, as well as the subjectively perceived health of a large sample of adults with congenital heart disease. The measurement of quality of life was built on a conceptual basis. Quality of life was defined and measured in terms of life satisfaction. This is in contrast to most quality of life reports, which measure quality of life as subjective health status. It has, however, been suggested that such an approach may be flawed, since quality of life and health status are two related, albeit distinct, concepts.[13,14] Indeed, the correlation between the linear analogue scale of quality of life and the linear analogue scale of health status in this study was 0.37 (95% confidence interval 0.30 to 0.44). Furthermore, a clear distinction was made between indicators (linear analogue scale, satisfaction with life scale) and determinants (SEIQoLDW) of quality of life. An appropriate assessment of quality of life needs to include one or more indicators of quality of life itself and may not be limited to the measurement of possible influential factors such as physical functioning, symptoms, perceived health, and mood.

We found a weak, negative association between the severity of congenital heart disease, quality of life, and perceived health. Results showed that heart disease severity had a detrimental impact on patients' lives only when it was measured in terms of poor functional status. This means that the initial diagnosis or the course of the illness does not influence quality of life or perceived health. The finding that correlations between functional status parameters and quality of life or perceived health were low indicates that patients with more severe conditions do not experience the congenital heart disease having a major effect on the overall perception of their life situation.

The achievement of optimal ventricular function has traditionally been the mainstay of outpatient and inpatient treatment for patients with congenital heart disease. This is largely based on the assumption that quality of life will follow ventricular performance. The present study refutes this assumption, as no significant associations were found between left ventricular ejection fraction and quality of life or health status. Note, however, that data on left ventricular function were excluded for patients with a transposition of the great arteries who had undergone an atrial switch repair (Mustard or Senning), since the right ventricle is the systemic ventricle in these patients.

Comparison with the literature
Empirical evidence on the relation between the severity of congenital heart disease and quality of life or subjective health status is scarce.[6-8,37] Using different conceptualizations and methods impedes the comparability of the results. Nonetheless, some similarities can be observed. Ternestedt and colleagues[7] found that patients with tetralogy of Fallot rated their quality of life higher than patients with atrial septal defect. This indicates that more severe heart defects are not necessarily associated with worse quality of life. Furthermore, no association between quality of life and NYHA class was found.[7]

This study confirmed the findings of Lane and colleagues[6] that subjective health status in patients with cyanotic conditions is lower than in those with acyanotic conditions.

The correlations between perceived health status and NYHA and between health status and ability index were also found by Kamphuis and colleagues.[8] Correlation coefficients cannot, however, be directly compared because Kamphuis and colleagues used the 36 item short form health survey (SF-36) and we used the linear analogue scale to assess perceived health status.

The present study was also in line with the results of a series of articles published by Meijboom and colleagues. Their studies in patients with atrial septal defect,[11] ventricular septal defect,[10] tetralogy of Fallot,[9] and transposition of the great arteries[12] indicated that subjectively perceived health status in the four diagnostic categories was fairly even.

Methodological limitations
In the absence of a de facto standard for the classification of the severity of congenital heart defects, various indicators of congenital heart disease severity were explored: initial medical diagnosis, the course of the illness, and functional status. The different angles of the respective classification systems are expressed by the disparities in frequency distribution (**table 2**) and by the limited interrelation. The validity of the classification schemes for use in quality of life research is uncertain. Only NYHA class and the ability index have previously been used in quality of life studies of congenital heart disease. Although the NYHA functional class is often used in clinical research on congenital heart disease, it purports to categorize patients with heart failure. If the classification system is merely based on the content of the NYHA class then it cannot be considered a valid tool for the categorization of patients with heart defects. Nonetheless, the NYHA class was consistently associated with quality of life and health status. Regarding the congenital heart disease functional index, no evidence on reliability and validity is available to date. Interrater variability was precluded since classification schemes were filled out by one cardiologist. Although a prognosis of life expectancy may also reflect the severity of a disease, this component was not included in this study, since individual prognosis cannot be predicted. Certain patients with congenital heart disease die of sudden death. So far, the risk of sudden death cannot be stratified.

The ideal means of assessing overall clinical and functional status is cardiopulmonary exercise testing, including the measurement of peak oxygen uptake. We did not include such exercise testing in the present study, which can be considered a methodological limitation. However, in a related study, we explored the association between maximum exercise capacity and peak oxygen uptake versus quality of life and self-perceived health in a sample of 36 patients with tetralogy of Fallot or transposition of the great arteries. Both quality of life and perceived health were not significantly related to maximum exercise capacity and peak oxygen uptake, with correlation coefficients ranging from 0.06–0.26 (data on file). These findings should, however, be interpreted with a measure of caution because of the very small sample size. Therefore, we did not include these results in the present chapter.

Although the sample of this study was large, it is not necessarily representative of the population of patients with congenital heart disease. This is because the eligible patients were recruited from the outpatient clinic of our center. It should be noted that many patients born with heart defects are treated in the first years of life and do not need regular follow up care at a tertiary care center. Patients with mild congenital heart diseases were underrepresented in this sample (26.1%), whereas this group accounts for 51% of the congenital heart disease population.[38] However, whether this underrepresentation has affected the results of this study is doubtful, since the severity of the congenital heart disease, in terms of initial diagnosis, does not influence patients' quality of life or perceived health. Furthermore, we did not include patients with mental retardation. Although inclusion of this group of patients would be of the utmost relevance, because they may be regarded as the most severely handicapped, they were excluded because self report by questionnaires requires intact intellectual abilities.

In this study, we evaluated only linear relations. Future research should therefore also investigate non-linear associations.

Recently, a disease specific instrument for adults with congenital heart disease was developed: congenital heart disease-TNO/AZL adult quality of life (CHD-TAAQOL).[39] Although we used this instrument in our sample,[28] we did not use it to assess the relation with disease severity because the CHD-TAAQOL does not result in a single aggregate score.

Conclusion

This study showed that the severity of congenital heart disease is marginally associated with patients' quality of life. Patients' assessment of their quality of life relates more to functional status than to the initial diagnosis or the course of the illness. Stronger associations were found between perceived health and functional status. Patients with cyanotic heart defects had lower perceptions of the status of their health than did acyanotic patients. The findings of this study are crucial to the development of key strategies to enhance the quality of life of this patient population and to provide appropriate counseling.

REFERENCES

1. Warnes CA, Liberthson R, Danielson GK, et al. Task force 1: the changing profile of congenital heart disease in adult life. J Am Coll Cardiol 2001;37:1170-5.
2. Meberg A, Otterstad JE, Froland G, et al. Outcome of congenital heart defects: a population-based study. Acta Paediatr 2000;89:1344-51.
3. Moons P, De Geest S, Budts W. Comprehensive care for adults with congenital heart disease: expanding roles for nurses. Eur J Cardiovasc Nurs 2002;1:23-8.
4. Strauss AL, Corbin J, Fagerhaugh S, et al. Chronic illness and the quality of life, 2nd ed.St. Louis: CV Mosby, 1984.
5. Walter PJ, Mohan R, Dahan-Mizrahl S. Quality of life after open heart surgery 16-18 May 1991. Qual Life Res 1992;1:77-83.
6. Lane DA, Lip GY, Millane TA. Quality of life in adults with congenital heart disease. Heart 2002;88:71-5.
7. Ternestedt BM, Wall K, Oddsson H, et al. Quality of life 20 and 30 years after surgery in patients operated on for tetralogy of Fallot and for atrial septal defect. Pediatr Cardiol 2001;22:128-32.
8. Kamphuis M, Ottenkamp J, Vliegen HW, et al. Health related quality of life and health status in adult survivors with previously operated complex congenital heart disease. Heart 2002;87:356-62.
9. Meijboom F, Szatmari A, Deckers JW, et al. Cardiac status and health-related quality of life in the long term after surgical repair of tetralogy of Fallot in infancy and childhood. J Thorac Cardiovasc Surg 1995;110:883-91.
10. Meijboom F, Szatmari A, Utens E, et al. Long-term follow-up after surgical closure of ventricular septal defect in infancy and childhood. J Am Coll Cardiol 1994;24:1358-64.
11. Meijboom F, Hess J, Szatmari A, et al. Long-term follow-up (9 to 20 years) after surgical closure of atrial septal defect at a young age. Am J Cardiol 1993;72:1431-4.
12. Meijboom F, Szatmari A, Deckers JW, et al. Long-term follow-up (10 to 17 years) after Mustard repair for transposition of the great arteries. J Thorac Cardiovasc Surg 1996;111:1158-68.
13. Smith KW, Avis NE, Assmann SF. Distinguishing between quality of life and health status in quality of life research: a meta-analysis. Qual Life Res 1999;8:447-59.
14. Bradley C. Importance of differentiating health status from quality of life. Lancet 2001;357:7-8.
15. Miller MR, Forrest CB, Kan JS. Parental preferences for primary and specialty care collaboration in the management of teenagers with congenital heart disease. Pediatrics 2000;106:264-9.
16. The Criteria Committee of the New York Heart Association. Nomenclature and criteria for diagnosis of diseases of the heart and great vessels, 9th ed. Boston: Little, Brown, 1994:253-6.
17. Somerville J. 'Grown-up' survivors of congenital heart disease: who knows? Who cares? Br J Hosp Med 1990;43:132-6.
18. Moons P, Siebens K, De Geest S, et al. A pilot study of expenditures on, and utilization of resources in, health care in adults with congenital heart disease. Cardiol Young 2001;11:301-13.
19. Gill TM, Feinstein AR. A critical appraisal of the quality of quality-of-life measurements. JAMA 1994;272:619-26.
20. Meeberg GA. Quality of life: a concept analysis. J Adv Nurs 1993;18:32-8. 21 Zhan L. Quality of life: conceptual and measurement issues. J Adv Nurs 1992;17:795-800.
22. Ferrans CE. Development of a conceptual model of quality of life. Sch Inq Nurs Pract 1996;10:293-304.
23. Jacobsen PB, Weitzner MA. Evaluation of palliative endpoints in oncology clinical trials. Cancer Control 1999;6:471-7.
24. de Boer AG, van Lanschot JJ, Stalmeier PF, et al. Is a single-item visual analogue scale as valid, reliable and responsive as multi-item scales in measuring quality of life? Qual Life Res 2004;13:311-20.

25. Fayers PM, Machin D. Quality of life: assessment, analysis and interpretation. Chichester: John Wiley and Sons, 2000.
26. Cunny KA, Perri M III. Single-item vs multiple-item measures of health-related quality of life. Psychol Rep 1991;69:127–30.
27. Michael M, Tannock IF. Measuring health-related quality of life in clinical trials that evaluate the role of chemotherapy in cancer treatment. CMAJ 1998;158:1727–34.
28. Moons P. Quality of life in adults with congenital heart disease: beyond the quantity of life. Leuven: P Moons, 2004, 1–165.
29. Diener E, Emmons RA, Larsen RJ, et al. The satisfaction with life scale. J Pers Soc Psychol 1985;49:71–5.
30. Pavot W, Diener E. Review of the satisfaction with life scale. Psychol Assess 1993;5:164–72.
31. Browne JP, O'Boyle CA, McGee HM, et al. Development of a direct weighting procedure for quality of life domains. Qual Life Res 1997;6:301–9.
32. Hickey AM, Bury G, O'Boyle CA, et al. A new short form individual quality of life measure (SEIQoL-DW): application in a cohort of individuals with HIV/AIDS. BMJ 1996;313:29–33.
33. Moons P, Marquet K, Budts W, et al. Validity, reliability and responsiveness of the "schedule for the evaluation of individual quality of life-direct weighting" (SEIQoL-DW) in congenital heart disease. Health Qual Life Outcomes 2004;2:27.
34. Badia X, Monserrat S, Roset M, et al. Feasibility, validity and test-retest reliability of scaling methods for health states: the visual analogue scale and the time trade-off. Qual Life Res 1999;8:303–10.
35. Sermeus W, Delesie L. Ridit analysis on ordinal data. West J Nurs Res 1996;18:351–9.
36. Cohen J. Statistical power analysis for the behavioral sciences. Hillsdale: Lawrence Erlbaum, 1988.
37. Walker WT, Temple IK, Gnanapragasam JP, et al. Quality of life after repair of tetralogy of Fallot. Cardiol Young 2002;12:549–53.
38. Hoffman JI, Kaplan S, Liberthson RR. Prevalence of congenital heart disease. Am Heart J 2004;147:425–39.
39. Kamphuis M, Zwinderman KH, Vogels T, et al. A cardiac-specific healthrelated quality of life module for young adults with congenital heart disease: development and validation. Qual Life Res 2004;13:735–45.

Chapter 6

Profile of adults with congenital heart disease having a good, moderate, or poor quality of life

Congenital heart defects are the most common birth defects and occur at a rate of approximately 8 in 1000 births [1]. It comprises a wide spectrum of simple, moderate, and complex severity lesions [2,3]. Because of advances in pediatric and interventional cardiology, in intensive care medicine, and in cardiac surgery, the number of children with congenital heart disease surviving into adulthood has continuously increased. As a consequence of higher survival rates, the prevalence of adults with congenital heart disease (ACHD) has increased as well. The number of ACHD patients in the population has been estimated to be approximately 5000 patients per million inhabitants [2,4]. For the first time in history, there are now more adults than children living with congenital heart defects, and this population is growing by approximately 5% per year [5].

Due to the increased life expectancy of children with congenital heart disease, the main focus of congenital cardiology care has shifted from survival towards long-term functioning. This shift has elicited heightened interest in quality-of-life issues in these patients. As a result, the number of publications on quality of life in children, adolescents, and adults with congenital heart disease has increased exponentially [6]. Some of these studies compared the quality of life of adult patients with that of the general population or with normative data [7-21]. In general, previous studies found that adult patients' quality of life is equivalent to that of the general population. When quality of life is measured in terms of functional status, scores of patient groups are lower than those of normative groups [14-17,19,21]. Conversely, one study found that patients with mild heart defects showed a better quality of life, if they did not present with social restrictions [7]. However, these studies had conspicuous methodological differences. Quality of life was either measured in terms of subjectively perceived health status [9-12], or by using the SF-36 [15,20,21]; the TAAQOL [7,14]; the Duke questionnaire [13]; the Sickness Impact Profile [16]; or the WHOQOL-Bref [19]. Other studies measured assorted variables considered either to be or to impact quality-of-life issues, such as health and medical history, marital and family life, educational attainment, insurability, and employability [8,18].

Despite the increasing interest in quality of life, consensus is lacking on the definition of quality of life. Quality of life is often used as a generic label to describe an assortment of physical and psychosocial variables. Therefore, quality of life often seems to be an umbrella term [22], covering a variety of concepts, such as functioning, health status, perceptions, life conditions, behavior, happiness, lifestyle, symptoms, etc. [23]. The absence of a uniform definition makes quality of life to be an ambiguous concept.

Over the past decade, several concept analyses of quality of life have been published [24-31]. More recently, we identified some critical conceptual problems and clarifications with regard to quality of life [32] (see chapter 2). Prior concept analyses along with the conceptual problems that we identified indicate that quality of life should be defined and measured in terms of life satisfaction. Accordingly, we defined quality of life as the degree of overall life satisfaction that is positively or negatively influenced by individuals' perception of certain aspects of life important to them, including matters both related and unrelated to health [33].

In a previous study, in which we measured quality of life in terms of life satisfaction in 629 adults with congenital heart disease, we found that patients reported overall a significantly better quality of life than matched healthy control subjects [34] (see chapter 3). This means that, although some patients do indeed experience a diminished quality of life, quality of life in patients with congenital heart disease is not necessarily poor. It is important to identify patients at risk for developing a poor quality of life. To date, no studies have been undertaken to investigate the differences in the characteristics of patients with a good or poor quality of life. The purpose of this study was therefore to assess the profile of adult patients with congenital heart disease who reported a good, moderate, or poor quality of life.

METHODS

Study population
We conducted a secondary analysis on data from a large-scale quality-of-life study, in which 629 adults with congenital heart disease were included [33-36]. Patients were enrolled from the outpatient clinic of our ACHD program. Criteria for inclusion were the following: 18 years of age or older; literate; Dutch speaking; and provided informed consent. Patients visiting our outpatient clinic for the first time, exhibiting mental retardation, or diagnosed with an atrial septal defect or a patent foramen ovale after cryptogenic stroke were excluded from the study. A detailed description of the selection procedure was previously reported [34]. Patients completed questionnaires after their scheduled visit at the outpatient clinic. The overall data collection procedure lasted approximately 15 to 20 min. Verbal informed consent was obtained from all participants.

Variables and measurements
Demographic and clinical information were retrieved from medical records and the hospital information system. Demographics included gender, age, educational level, employment status, and marital status. Clinical variables included primary diagnosis; current and past treatment (current medication intake, as well as previous operations, catheter interventions, electrophysiological treatments); heredity of the heart defect; presence of associated syndromes; stability of the heart defect; and complications. Data on functional status, expressed in terms of New York Heart Association (NYHA) functional classes, were provided by the cardiologist, based on information from the patient interview.

A Linear Analogue Scale (LAS) was employed to assess quality of life. The LAS consisted of a vertically oriented, 10-centimeter line, graded with indicators ranging from 0 (worst imaginable quality of life) to 100 (best imaginable quality of life). Respondents were asked to rate their overall quality of life by marking the point on the scale that corresponded to how good or bad their present quality of life was. The psychometric properties of the LAS for use in adults with congenital heart disease have been evaluated, and were detailed in a previous article [34]. Evidence based on test content, evidence based on relation with other variables, evidence on reliability, and evidence on responsiveness were provided, and showed that the LAS is valid, reliable, and responsive for its purpose [34].

Data analysis
The computer program Statistical Package of the Social Sciences 12.0 (SPSS™; SPSS Inc., Chicago, Illinois) was used to analyze the data. Descriptive statistics were expressed in absolute numbers and percentages for nominal level data, and in medians and quartiles (Q1 and Q3) for continuous variables, because they were not normally distributed. We used K-means cluster analysis to empirically classify patients according to their quality of life. Cluster analysis aims to partition subjects into different groups on the basis of a minimal within-group and a maximal between-group variation [37]. The algorithm in K-means cluster analysis requires the a priori definition of the number of clusters. On the basis of the quality-of-life scores on the LAS, we categorized patients into a 3-cluster solution: good, moderate, or poor quality of life. Statistical differences between the groups were investigated using the Chi-square test and the Kruskal–Wallis test for nominal and continuous independent variables, respectively. If the assumptions for the Chi-square test were not fulfilled, the Fisher's Exact test was computed.

Since multiple tests were performed, we accounted for the multiple testing phenomenon by using the false discovery rate method of Benjamini [38]. With this approach, the expected number of type I errors were kept below 5%, and the adjusted p-values were denoted as q-values. A q-value of 0.05 was considered statistically significant.

Results

Sample characteristics
The sample consisted of 629 adults with congenital heart disease. Two patients did not complete the LAS for quality of life. Hence, the analysis pertains to 627 patients, 378 (60.3%) of which were male. The median age was 24 years (Q1=20; Q3=29). This relatively young age implies that the majority of the patients was unmarried and living with their parents (55.4%). In this sample, 27.9% were students and 59.8% were employed as blue-collar workers, white-collar workers, or were self-employed. The most prevalent heart defects were tetralogy of Fallot, ventricular septal defect, coarctation of the aorta, congenital stenosis of the aortic valve, pulmonary valve stenosis, and complete transposition of the great arteries (**Table 1**).

Quality of life
The analysis clustered 490 patients (78.1%) into the group having a good quality of life; 126 patients (20.1%) having a moderate quality of life; and 11 patients (1.8%) having a poor quality of life. In **Figure 1**, a box plot of quality-of-life scores according to cluster membership is given.

Figure 1: Box plot of quality-of-life scores in 627 adults with congenital heart disease according to cluster membership

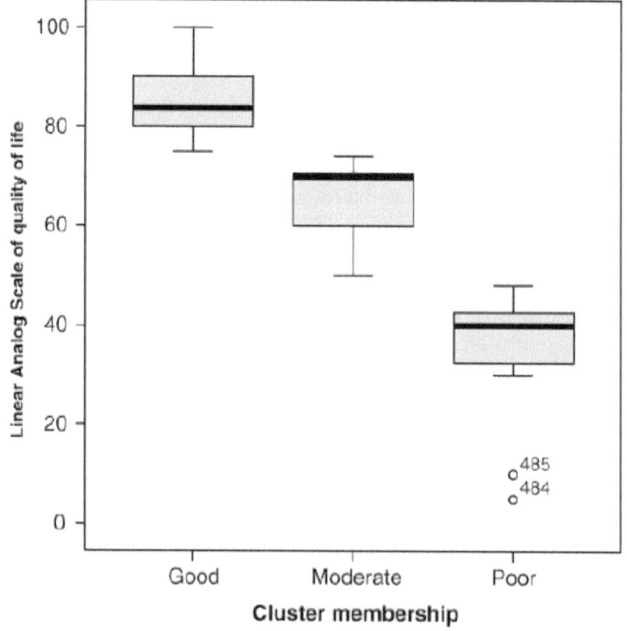

The demographic and clinical characteristics for which a significant difference was found among the quality-of-life clusters were educational level, employment status, associated syndromes, stability of the heart defect, and NYHA classification (**Table 1**). The group of patients with a good quality of life appeared to have a higher educational level than the other groups of patients. Patients categorized as having a good quality of life more often had a college or university degree than patients categorized as having a moderate quality of life. Vocational high school was more frequently associated with patients in the moderate or poor quality-of-life cluster than with patients in the good quality-of-life cluster. In terms of employment status, patients who were unemployed or disabled more frequently had a moderate or poor quality of life. By contrast, students were more likely to report a good quality of life.

With respect to the clinical variables, we observed that the proportion of patients with associated syndromes was the highest in the moderate quality-of-life cluster. Patients with an unstable heart condition and patients with a worse NYHA functional class reported a poorer quality of life, with the highest proportion in the poor quality-of-life cluster.

Gender, age, marital status, primary heart defect, mode of treatment, complications, and inherited heart defect were not significantly associated with quality of life.

Discussion

Previous studies have found that the quality of life of ACHD patients is basically equivalent to that of the general population. Some studies have indicated that patients' quality of life can be even better than that of healthy peers [7,34]. It is, however, important to know which patients are vulnerable to developing a poor quality of life. Therefore, we undertook a cluster analytic study to assess the profile of adult patients with congenital heart disease who reported a good, moderate, or poor quality of life. The results of this study can be used to identify vulnerable patients who might benefit from specific interventions that can help them avoid a diminished quality of life. Such interventions can be performed by nurse specialists involved in ACHD care [39,40].

Three-quarters of the patients had a good quality of life, one-fifth had a moderate quality of life, and only a small minority had a poor quality of life. Given the fact that congenital heart disease can be considered to be a chronic condition in many patients, it might be surprising that they report such a good quality of life. Possible pathways explaining why patients

Table 1 Demographic and clinical characteristics of 627 adult patients with congenital heart disease according to cluster membership

Variable	Overall sample	Good quality of life	Moderate quality of life	Poor quality of life	Test; q-value
Gender: (n=627)					Chi^2=2.584; q=0.302
Male	378 (60.3%)	301 (61.4%)	69 (54.8%)	8 (72.7%)	
Female	249 (39.7%)	189 (38.6%)	57 (45.2%)	3 (27.3%)	
Median age (years): (n=627)	24 (Q_1=20; Q_3=29)	23 (Q_1=20; Q_3=28)	24 (Q_1=20; Q_3=32)	30 (Q_1=20; Q_3=45)	Chi^2=2.370#; q=0.306
	range 18 – 66	range 18 – 66	range 18 – 55	range 18 – 55	
Marital status: (n=624)					Chi^2=7.203; q=0.189
Unmarried (living with parents)	346 (55.4%)	268 (55.0%)	75 (59.5%)	3 (27.3%)	
Living alone, divorced, or widowed	59 (9.5%)	43 (8.8%)	15 (11.9%)	1 (9.1%)	
Married or cohabitating	219 (35.1%)	176 (36.2%)	36 (28.6%)	7 (63.6%)	
Highest educational level: (n=619)					F.E.=23.76; q=0.042
Primary education	3 (0.5%)	3 (0.6%)	0 (0.0%)	0 (0.0%)	
Special needs education	11 (1.8%)	6 (1.2%)	5 (4.0%)	0 (0.0%)	
Vocational high school	215 (34.7%)	151 (31.3%)	60 (47.6%)	4 (40.0%)	
Technical high school	81 (13.1%)	66 (13.7%)	13 (10.3%)	2 (20.0%)	
High school	52 (8.4%)	39 (8.1%)	13 (10.3%)	0 (0.0%)	
College	175 (28.3%)	149 (30.8%)	24 (19.1%)	2 (20.0%)	
University	82 (13.2%)	69 (14.3%)	11 (8.7%)	2 (20.0%)	
Employment status (n=627)					F.E.=20.944; q=0.042
Student	175 (27.9%)	147 (30.0%)	26 (20.6%)	2 (18.2%)	
Employed	375 (59.8%)	294 (60.0%)	73 (57.9%)	8 (72.7%)	
Unemployed/Looking for work	37 (5.9%)	24 (4.9%)	13 (10.3%)	0 (0.0%)	
Unable to work/Disability	16 (2.6%)	8 (1.6%)	7 (5.6%)	1 (9.1%)	
Retired	5 (0.8%)	5 (1.0%)	0 (0.0%)	0 (0.0%)	
Other	19 (3.0%)	12 (2.5%)	7 (5.6%)	0 (0.0%)	
Primary medical diagnosis: (n=627)					F.E.=12.96; q=0.302
Tetralogy of Fallot	111 (17.7%)	80 (16.3%)	29 (23.0%)	2 (18.2%)	
Ventricular Septal Defect (VSD)	108 (17.2%)	92 (18.8%)	15 (11.9%)	1 (9.1%)	
Coarctation of the aorta	89 (14.2%)	75 (15.3%)	13 (10.3%)	1 (9.1%)	
Congenital stenosis of aortic valve	65 (10.4%)	47 (9.6%)	16 (12.7%)	2 (18.2%)	
Pulmonary valve stenosis (congenital)	48 (7.7%)	36 (7.4%)	11 (8.7%)	1 (9.1%)	
Complete transposition of great vessels	36 (5.7%)	32 (6.5%)	4 (3.2%)	0 (0.0%)	
Other	170 (27.1%)	128 (26.1%)	38 (30.2%)	4 (36.3%)	

Treatment (n=627)				
Surgery	397 (63.3%)	299 (61.0%)	10 (90.9%)	Chi²=7.027; q=0.064
Catheter intervention	96 (15.3%)	69 (14.1%)	2 (18.2%)	Chi²=2.635; q=0.302
Medication	106 (16.9%)	73 (14.9%)	3 (27.3%)	Chi²=6.523; q=0.071
AICD/reconversion/pacemaker	49 (7.8%)	35 (7.1%)	0 (0.0%)	Chi²=3.140; q=0.284
Hereditary of the heart defect: (n=626)				F.E.=7.636; q=0.143
Yes	29 (4.6%)	17 (3.5%)	0 (0.0%)	
No	580 (92.7%)	459 (93.9%)	11 (100.0%)	
Unsure	17 (2.7%)	13 (2.6%)	0 (0.0%)	
Associated syndromes: (n=625)				Chi²=8.522; q=0.042
Yes	26 (4.2%)	15 (3.1%)	0 (0.0%)	
No	599 (95.8%)	473 (96.9%)	11 (100%)	
Stability of the heart defect: (n=626)				Chi²=14.585; q=0.008
Yes	599 (95.7%)	471 (96.3%)	8 (72.7%)	
No	27 (4.3%)	18 (3.7%)	3 (27.3%)	
Having had complications: (n=542)				Chi²=6.987; q=0.064
Yes	139 (25.6%)	100 (23.4%)	5 (50.0%)	
No	403 (74.4%)	328 (76.6%)	5 (50.0%)	
New York Heart Association functional class: (n=625)				F.E.=27.142; q=0.008
Class I	511 (81.7%)	419 (85.7%)	6 (54.5%)	
Class II	83 (13.3%)	52 (10.6%)	3 (27.3%)	
Class III	26 (4.2%)	14 (2.9%)	2 (18.2%)	
Class IV	5 (0.8%)	4 (0.8%)	0 (0.0%)	

F.E. = Fisher's Exact test for M * N tables; # = Kruskal Wallis test with heart defects experience a considerably good quality of life are the (i) disability paradox [41]; (ii) sense of coherence [42]; and (iii) response shift [43]. These issues have been described in detail in chapter 3.

Factors associated with quality of life
In the present study, we observed factors that were associated with patients' quality of life. Characteristics that were associated with a poorer quality of life (moderate or poor quality-of-life clusters) were a lower educational level, being unemployed or disabled, having associated syndromes, instability of the heart disease, and a poorer functional status. To our knowledge, this is the first investigation comparing demographic and clinical characteristics of ACHD patients in terms of different levels of quality of life. Therefore, the findings of our study cannot be compared with those of previous reports. Nonetheless, some investigations have tried to assess determinants of quality of life in ACHD [13,18,19]. However, these studies provided descriptions of different dimensions of health status rather than single quality-of-life index scores, or they focused on operative determinants of specific heart lesions rather than on demographic or long-term follow-up data of the overall population.

It was not surprising that patients with an unstable medical condition and with a reduced functional status had a poorer quality of life. Indeed, these aspects represent a poor medical status. It was also not surprising that the primary diagnosis did not differ among the three groups, since we previously reported that quality of life in ACHD is only marginally associated with the severity of the heart defect [36]. However, our findings with respect to age and gender were not in line with our expectations. In general, quality of life research on cardiovascular populations shows that gender differences exist, with women basically having a lower quality of life than men [44]. Moreover, quality of life scores alter when patients grow older [45]. A literature review on quality of life in older patient populations revealed that quality of life in older persons is considerably lower than that of younger age groups, if quality of life is phrased in relation to the person's physical functioning [45]. When older people are asked to report on their health status, they tend to perceiving their health significantly more positively than younger people; and considering themselves to be healthier than their peers [45]. This is thought to be related to different expectations regarding health and functional status. In the present study, we did not corroborate this relationship between age/gender and quality of life, illustrating that adults with congenital heart disease constitute a specific patient group, one different from other cardiovascular populations.

Methodological issues

When interpreting the results of this secondary data analysis, we should bear in mind some methodological limitations inherent to the original study. One limitation was that the respondents were recruited at the outpatient clinic of the ACHD program. Therefore, the sample is not necessarily representative of the entire population of patients with cardiac anomalies [34]. A second limitation was that the study was conducted at a single centre, thus compromising the generalizability of our results towards larger populations of patients with congenital heart disease [34]. A third limitation was that we excluded patients with significant developmental delays from participating in our study, even though including these patients would have been very relevant to our study, since developmentally delayed patients can be considered to be the most severely handicapped patients. We excluded these patients because filling-out the questionnaires used in this study requires intact intellectual abilities [34].

For our secondary data analysis, we computed 15 statistical tests. We corrected for the multiple testing phenomenon by using a q-value instead of the traditional p-value. However, in order to limit the inflating of type I error, we did not conduct post hoc tests to investigate which specific groups differed statistically. Nonetheless, descriptive statistics could assist us in determining where the differences existed.

Some studies reported in the literature make use of quartiles of quality-of-life scores to categorize patients into different groups. In our study, we used K-means cluster analysis. We believe that this approach is empirically sounder. However, this has resulted in unbalanced subgroups, implying that exact tests were required in some analyses. The unbalanced subgroups also made it impossible to perform multivariate analyses. During the analysis process, we performed multinomial logistic regression. However, due to the small group of patients with a poor quality of life, the validity of the model fit was uncertain. Therefore, we limited the reported results to those obtained with the bivariate analyses.

This study provides a basis for a sequential quan–qual design [46]. Indeed, it would be very interesting to obtain more in-depth information on why patients consider their quality of life to be good, moderate, or poor. Cluster membership, as found in the present study, could be used to approach some patients from each cluster to participate in a qualitative study, using in-depth interviews. A mixed method approach of quantitative and qualitative research designs has been reported to be most valuable [50].

CONCLUSIONS

In this study, we investigated the profile of adults with congenital heart disease who reported a good, moderate, or poor quality of life. Three-quarters of the patients had a good quality of life, whereas only a small minority could be considered to have a poor quality of life. Patients with a poorer quality of life were characterized by a lower educational level, being unemployed or disabled, having associated syndromes, instability of the heart disease, and a poorer functional status as measured by the NYHA classification scheme. The findings of this study can be used to identify patients who are prone to developing a poor quality of life. Specific nursing interventions that support these vulnerable patients can be applied in order to avoid a diminished quality of life.

REFERENCES

1. Hoffman JI, Kaplan S. The incidence of congenital heart disease. J Am Coll Cardiol 2002;39:1890-900.
2. Hoffman JI, Kaplan S, Liberthson RR. Prevalence of congenital heart disease. Am Heart J 2004;147:425-39.
3. Warnes CA, Liberthson R, Danielson GK, Dore A, Harris L, Hoffman JI, et al. Task force 1: the changing profile of congenital heart disease in adult life. J Am Coll Cardiol 2001;37:1170-5.
4. Marelli AJ, Mackie AS, Ionescu-Ittu R, Rahme E, Pilote L. Congenital heart disease in the general population: changing prevalence and age distribution. Circulation 2007;115:163-72.
5. Brickner ME, Hillis LD, Lange RA. Congenital heart disease in adults. First of two parts. N Engl J Med 2000;342:256-63.
6. Moons P, Van Deyk K, BudtsW, De Geest S. Caliber of quality-of-life assessments in congenital heart disease: a plea for more conceptual and methodological rigor. Arch Pediatr Adolesc Med 2004;158:1062-9.
7. Fekkes M, Kamphuis RP, Ottenkamp J, Verrips E, Vogels T, Kamphuis M, et al. Health-related quality of life in young adults with minor congenital heart disease. Psychol Health 2001;16:239-50.
8. Gersony WM, Hayes CJ, Driscoll DJ, Keane JF, Kidd L, O'Fallon WM, et al. Second natural history study of congenital heart defects. Quality of life of patients with aortic stenosis, pulmonary stenosis, or ventricular septal defect. Circulation 1993;87:I52-65.
9. Meijboom F, Hess J, Szatmari A, Utens EM, McGhie J, Deckers JW, et al. Long-term follow-up (9 to 20 years) after surgical closure of atrial septal defect at a young age. Am J Cardiol 1993;72:1431-4.
10. Meijboom F, Szatmari A, Utens E, Deckers JW, Roelandt JR, Bos E, et al. Long-term follow-up after surgical closure of ventricular septal defect in infancy and childhood. J Am Coll Cardiol 1994;24:1358-64.
11. Meijboom F, Szatmari A, Deckers JW, Utens EM, Roelandt JR, Bos E, et al. Cardiac status and health-related quality of life in the long term after surgical repair of tetralogy of Fallot in infancy and childhood. J Thorac Cardiovasc Surg 1995;110:883-91.
12. Meijboom F, Szatmari A, Deckers JW, Utens EM, Roelandt JR, Bos E, et al. Long-term follow-up (10 to 17 years) after Mustard repair for transposition of the great arteries. J Thorac Cardiovasc Surg 1996;111:1158-68.
13. Saliba Z, Butera G, Bonnet D, Bonhoeffer P, Villain E, Kachaner J, et al. Quality of life and perceived health status in surviving adults with univentricular heart. Heart 2001;86:69-73.

14. Kamphuis M, Ottenkamp J, Vliegen HW, Vogels T, Zwinderman KH, Kamphuis RP, et al. Health related quality of life and health status in adult survivors with previously operated complex congenital heart disease. Heart 2002;87:356-62.
15. Lane DA, Lip GY, Millane TA. Quality of life in adults with congenital heart disease. Heart 2002;88:71-5.
16. Simko LC, McGinnis KA. Quality of life experienced by adults with congenital heart disease. AACN Clin Issues 2003;14:42-53.
17. Simko LC, McGinnis KA. What is the perceived quality of life of adults with congenital heart disease and does it differ by anomaly? J Cardiovasc Nurs 2005;20:206-14.
18. Walker WT, Temple IK, Gnanapragasam JP, Goddard JR, Brown EM. Quality of life after repair of tetralogy of Fallot. Cardiol Young 2002;12:549-53.
19. Rose M, Kohler K, Kohler F, Sawitzky B, Fliege H, Klapp BF. Determinants of the quality of life of patients with congenital heart disease. Qual Life Res 2005;14:35-43.
20. Immer FF, Althaus SM, Berdat PA, Saner H, Carrel TP. Quality of life and specific problems after cardiac surgery in adolescents and adults with congenital heart diseases. Eur J Cardiovasc Prev Rehabil 2005;12:138-43.
21. Jefferies JL, Noonan JA, Keller BB, Wilson JF, Griffith III C. Quality of life and social outcomes in adults with congenital heart disease living in rural areas of Kentucky. Am J Cardiol 2004;94:263-6.
22. Feinstein AR. Clinimetric perspectives. J Chronic Dis 1987;40:635-40. [23] Simko LC. Adults with congenital heart disease: utilizing quality of life and Husted's nursing theory as a conceptual framework. Crit Care Nurs Q 1999;22:1-11.
24. MeebergGA.Quality of life: a concept analysis. JAdvNurs 1993;18:32-8.
25. Zhan L. Quality of life: conceptual and measurement issues. J Adv Nurs 1992;17:795-800.
26. Felce D. Defining and applying the concept of quality of life. J Intellect Disabil Res 1997;41(Pt 2):126-35.
27. Ferrans CE. Quality of life: conceptual issues. Semin Oncol Nurs 1990;6:248-54.
28. Haas BK. A multidisciplinary concept analysis of quality of life.West J Nurs Res 1999;21:728-42.
29. Haas BK. Clarification and integration of similar quality of life concepts. Image J Nurs Sch 1999;31:215-20.
30. Stewart A. Conceptual and methodologic issues in defining quality of life: state of the art. Prog Cardiovasc Nurs 1992;7:3-11.
31. Kleinpell RM. Concept analysis of quality of life. Dimens Crit Care Nurs 1991;10:223-9.
32. Moons P, Budts W, De Geest S. Critique on the conceptualisation of quality of life: a review and evaluation of different conceptual approaches. Int J Nurs Stud 2006;43:891-901.
33. Moons P, Marquet K, Budts W, De Geest S. Validity, reliability and responsiveness of the "Schedule for the Evaluation of Individual Quality of Life — Direct Weighting" (SEIQoL-DW) in congenital heart disease. Health Qual Life Outcomes 2004;2:27.
34. Moons P, Van Deyk K, De Bleser L, Marquet K, Raes E, De Geest S, et al. Quality of life and health status in adults with congenital heart disease: a direct comparison with healthy counterparts. Eur J Cardiovasc Prev Rehabil 2006;13:407-13.
35. Moons P, Van Deyk K, Marquet K, Raes E, De Bleser L, BudtsW, et al. Individual quality of life in adults with congenital heart disease: a paradigm shift. Eur Heart J 2005;26:298-307.
36. Moons P, Van Deyk K, De Geest S, Gewillig M, Budts W. Is the severity of congenital heart disease associated with the quality of life and perceived health of adult patients? Heart 2005;91:1193-8.
37. Steinley D. K-means clustering: a half-century synthesis. Br J Math Stat Psychol 2006;59:1-34.
38. BenjaminiY,HochbergY. Controlling the false discovery rate—a practical and powerful approach to multiple testing. J R Stat Soc Ser B Methodol 1995;57:289-300.
39. Moons P, De Geest S, Budts W. Comprehensive care for adults with congenital heart disease: expanding roles for nurses. Eur J Cardiovasc Nurs 2002;1:23-8.
40. Moons P, Scholte op Reimer W, De Geest S, Fridlund B, Heikkila J, Jaarsma T, et al. Nurse specialists in adult congenital heart disease: the current status in Europe. Eur J Cardiovasc Nurs 2006;5:60-7.

41. Albrecht GL, Devlieger PJ. The disability paradox: high quality of life against all odds. Soc Sci Med 1999;48:977–88.
42. Antonovsky A. Unraveling the mystery of health: how people manage stress and stay well. San Fransisco: Jossey-Bass; 1987.
43. Rapkin BD, Schwartz CE. Toward a theoretical model of quality-of-life appraisal: implications of findings from studies of response shift. Health Qual Life Outcomes 2004;2:14.
44. Pilote L, Dasgupta K, Guru V, Humphries KH, McGrath J, Norris C, et al. A comprehensive view of sex-specific issues related to cardiovascular disease. CMAJ 2007;176:S1–44.
45. Hickey A, Barker M, McGee H, O'Boyle C. Measuring health-related quality of life in older patient populations: a review of current approaches. Pharmacoeconomics 2005;23:971–93.
46. Tashakkori A, Teddlie C. Handbook of mixed methods in social and behavioral research. Thousand Oaks: Sage Publications; 2003.

Chapter 7

Sense of coherence as a pathway to explain why patients with congenital heart disease have a better quality of life

Due to advances in medicine, and in particular surgery, diseases formerly considered to be lethal have evolved into conditions now considered to be chronic. This has led to a dramatic increase in quality-of-life research. In addition to mortality, morbidity, satisfaction with care, and health-care costs, quality of life has become a key outcome parameter when evaluating health care provisions [1]. Indeed, an essential goal of health care or nursing interventions is to promote a favorable quality of life, prompting many to study the quality of life of specific patient populations and to assess the beneficial effects of dedicated interventions or therapeutic modes on patients' quality of life.

Recently, a quality-of-life study in adult patients with congenital heart disease sought to identify issues or domains that primarily affect these patients' quality of life [2-4] (see chapters 3, 4, 5). That study revealed that adult patients with congenital heart disease felt that they had a good quality of life, one that was better than that of healthy counterparts [4]. This finding was surprising, since previous studies comparing this patient group to the general population indicated that the quality of life of adults with congenital heart disease was equivalent to that of the general population [5-12]. Other studies indicated that these patients have a lower level of functioning than do control subjects, when quality of life was assessed with a functional status instrument [13-15]. Moreover, many consider congenital heart defects to be chronic conditions because many factors can interfere with everyday life of these patients, including the long-term nature of congenital heart disease, the uncertainty of illness course and prognosis, the signs and symptoms of the illness, and restrictions in activity level [16].

One particular concept that appears to be relevant to explain the better quality of life in adults with congenital heart disease is sense of coherence (SOC). The aims of this chapter are to detail why SOC could be one explanation for the better quality of life in adults with congenital heart disease measured by Moons [4], and advance the hypothesis that SOC is a means for improving the quality of life in patients who grow up with a chronic disease. We consider congenital heart disease as an exemplar for other chronic diseases.

QUALITY OF LIFE

Today, there is a lack of consensus regarding the conceptualization, operational definition, and measurement of quality of life. Quality of life is often incorrectly used as a generic label to describe a range of physical and psychosocial variables, making quality of life an umbrella term, covering a variety of concepts [17]. Over the past decade, several concept analyses of quality of life have been published [18-25]. In addition, we identified some critical conceptual pitfalls and clarifications with regard to quality of life (see chapter 2). Together with prior concept analyses, the evaluation of these pitfalls indicates that quality of life should be defined and measured in terms of life satisfaction. Accordingly, for the study in patients with congenital heart disease, quality of life was defined as the degree of overall life satisfaction that is positively or negatively influenced by individuals' perception of certain aspects of life important to them, including matters both related and unrelated to health [4].

SENSE OF COHERENCE

Antonovsky developed the concept of SOC to explain why some people become ill when stressed, whereas others remain healthy [26]. SOC is the central construct of Antonovsky's salutogenic model, which posits that, to create healthy wellbeing, it is more important for people to focus on their resources and capacities rather than to focus on their disease (i.e., the classic pathogenic perspective). SOC is defined as "a global orientation that expresses the extent to which one has a pervasive, enduring though dynamic feeling of confidence that (i) the stimuli deriving from one's internal and external environments in the course of living are structured, predictable, and explicable; (ii) the resources are available to one to meet the demands posed by these stimuli; and (iii) these demands are challenges, worthy of investment and engagement" [26]. Hence, SOC is a general expression of an individual's view of the world. It has three components: (i) comprehensibility, (ii) manageability, and (iii) meaningfulness. Elevated comprehensibility, manageability, and meaningfulness reflect a higher degree of SOC. Antonovsky argues that a strong SOC is crucial to coping with the many stressors of life, and consequently, to health maintenance [26]. Indeed, a basic assumption to maintain health is a person's ability to adapt to illness, with possible changes in the level of expectations and aspirations as a result. Numerous studies of diverse populations have shown that SOC is strongly associated with quality of life [27-40].

DEVELOPING SENSE OF COHERENCE

SOC develops during childhood and youth and is thought, based on theoretical considerations, to be fully developed by the age of 30 years [26]. SOC changes most during adolescence, because one has many choices and many areas of life are yet to be established. Unless radical changes in social or living conditions occur, SOC remains relatively stable after an individual reaches the age of 30 years [26,41]. This is especially the case for individuals with high SOCs. Recent findings suggest, however, that SOC tends to increase with age [42]. In addition, some findings suggest that disease progress or medical interventions may induce intrapersonal alterations of SOC [41,43-45].

Perceiving the availability of generalized resistance resources and having the ability to use them appears to be pivotal in developing a strong SOC [46]. Generalized resistance resources comprise a broad range of resources that neutralizes the effects of stressful life events and promotes successful tension management [46]. Examples include social support, childhood experiences, material resources, intelligence, coping strategies, family socialization, egoidentity, and physical characteristics [26,46]. There is a dynamic relationship between stressors and general resistance resources. Repeated exposure to various stressful events during life and the successful management of those events help an individual to develop generalized resistance resources, and consequently, to strengthen that individual's SOC [46]. In turn, a strong SOC can mobilize a person to apply his resistance resources as he seeks a solution to his problem or as he copes with a stressor [26,46]. These findings harmonize with the reciprocal relationship between SOC and generalized resistance resources [46].

GROWING UP WITH CONGENITAL HEART DISEASE

Since individuals with congenital heart disease are born with this condition, they develop mechanisms to cope with their condition at an early age, and they continue to develop and refine these mechanisms well into adulthood. This ability to cope may explain the findings of Moons and colleagues that adults with congenital heart disease generally view themselves as having a good quality of life [2-4]. In other words, patients were satisfied with the life they were living. Thus, we hypothesize that growing up with a congenital heart defect can positively influence SOC development, because congenital heart disease may be associated with a set of experiences that enhances comprehensibility, manageability, and meaningfulness. Because the health of children with congenital heart disease is monitored closely, health care professionals can also contribute significantly to the development of a strong SOC. Below, we discuss how growing up with congenital heart disease can influence SOC in relation to the three SOC components.

Comprehensibility

Comprehensibility is the extent by which the internal and external environmental stimuli one experiences during childhood are structured, predictable, and explainable [26]. Living with congenital heart disease can be stressful for a child, because both the complexity and uncertainty of the condition can initially overwhelm both child and parents. By educating the child about his disease, parents and health care professionals can make the condition more predictable for the child. In this respect, consistency is paramount in what parents and health care professionals teach the child about his disease [47].

While studying the lived experiences of adults with congenital heart disease, Claessens and colleagues found that parents who openly talk about the heart defect with their child instill in their child a realistic view of living with a heart disease [48]. Consequently, they prepare their child to realistically deal early on in life with limitations inherent to the disease. By contrast, parents who conceal the heart defect from their child (to protect their child from adverse experiences) instill in their child a false sense of security [48]. Consequently, they fail to prepare their child to deal with the disease, forcing the child to confront his limitations later on in life. Thus, parental overprotection during childhood can make it more difficult for individuals with congenital heart disease to successfully integrate their illness into daily life [48], because their parents prevented them from viewing their heart defect in a structured, predictable, and explainable way. Consequently, these individuals may view themselves as different from others that do not have the disease [48].

To promote SOC development, health care professionals ought to openly communicate the heart defect and its consequences with parents and children. Structured education programs are indispensable in this respect. Furthermore, they should encourage parents to give the heart defect a realistic place in their child's life. In this way, health care workers can serve as a generalized resistance resource, enhancing comprehensibility.

Children with congenital heart disease can have a more comprehensible life than do healthy children, because they explicitly discuss their concerns more often with their parents and health care workers. Thus, patients with congenital heart disease can be assumed to have an enhanced sense of comprehensibility and SOC.

Manageability

Manageability refers to the perceived resources that an individual has to manage stressful stimuli [26]. Experiences of an appropriate load balance determine manageability [47]. In other words, having too many or too few stressors hampers manageability development, because such experiences do not promote self-confidence in an individual. Therefore, for individuals with congenital heart disease, achieving balance between stressors (i.e., living with the heart defect) and perceived resources is important. One type of generalized resistance resource alluded to above is the supportive relationship a child has with his parents and health care professionals. These persons can make living with a heart defect less traumatic for a child. Health care workers can make their patients aware of other resistance resources by informing and encouraging them. When children feel they are competent to deal with the problems associated with their disease, they develop an increased sense of manageability, which in turn leads to a stronger SOC. Because healthy children do not have to deal with the stress of living with a chronic illness, they may have fewer opportunities to cultivate a strong sense of manageability.

Meaningfulness
Meaningfulness is the extent to which an individual believes that life makes sense emotionally. Meaningfulness also conveys the idea of one possessing the motivation and desire to cope with stimuli [26]. In this respect, it is important that an individual feels that he has control over his fate, rather than feeling that he is at the mercy of others. Hence, an individual develops heightened meaningfulness when he participates in shaping his future [46]. To promote the development of meaningfulness, it is critical that adults show children and adolescents that they are appreciated [26].

Individuals that have had surgery as treatment of their congenital heart defect often experience heightened existentialism. While qualitatively assessing the lived experiences of adults with congenital heart disease, Claessens and coworkers found that most patients viewed their cardiac surgery as a turning point in their lives [48]. Because surgery improves their physical capacity and enhances their appreciation for the "little things" in life, patients often divide their lives into two periods: before and after their operation. Such experiences can help patients find meaning in their lives and acknowledge that the demands placed on them by having congenital heart disease are worth their efforts. This experience builds up their sense of meaningfulness.

Parents and health care professionals can also help patients develop meaningfulness by supporting them as they try to take control of their lives, involving them in decision making. Again, healthy children may not have as many opportunities as do children with congenital heart disease to develop meaningfulness.

GAINING SENSE OF COHERENCE TO IMPROVE QUALITY OF LIFE

We previously stated that patients with congenital heart disease rate themselves as having a better quality of life than do healthy control subjects [4]. Our discussion of the elements above supports the hypothesis that patients with congenital heart disease could develop a stronger SOC than do healthy counterparts. We propose that an individual might be more likely to develop a strong SOC if (i) parents and health care workers educate that individual about his disease, giving them consistent information; (ii) they support that individual, making living with the disease as balanced as possible; and (iii) individuals view life threatening episodes as experiences that bring about meaning to their lives. Research is needed on SOC in adults with congenital heart disease to substantiate these ideas.

The SOC phenomenon also likely applies to children suffering from other types of chronic diseases, such as diabetes, asthma, cystic fibrosis, and renal failure, amongst others. These children have the potential for developing a strong SOC, as long as they do not perceive their disorders as too burdensome.

In summary, we advance the hypothesis that developing SOC can improve the quality of life of patients who grow up with a chronic disease, if quality of life is defined in terms of life satisfaction. This justifies the initiation of long-term longitudinal studies that examine SOC development in children with chronic diseases, how generalized resistance resources contribute to that development, and how SOC affects the quality of life of these children when they become adults. To date, most research has focused on SOC as a determinant of health or has investigated living conditions or family dynamics as factors influencing SOC development [46]. The relationship between chronic illness in childhood and SOC development is yet to be studied. We argue that these issues should be put on the research agenda.

If empirical evidence confirms that living with a chronic disorder in childhood enhances strong SOC development, this can greatly broaden nurses' roles in caring for children with chronic illnesses. To help these children develop a strong SOC, as nurses we will need to educate children about their illness, help children balance the stresses of their diseases, and encourage children to participate in any decisions dealing with the management of their disease. We will also need to encourage parents to do the same. SOC can be an important target for interventions in childhood to improve patients' quality of life during adulthood.

REFERENCES

1. Radosevich DM, Kalambokidis Werni TL. Using outcomes measures to assess the quality of health care. In: Radosevich DM, Kalambokidis Werni TL, editors. A practical guidebook for implementing, analyzing, and reporting outcomes measurements. Bloomington' Health Outcomes Institute, 1996. p. 1 -10.
2. Moons P, Van Deyk K, Marquet K, Raes E, De Bleser L, Budts W, et al. Individual quality of life in adults with congenital heart disease: a paradigm shift. Eur Heart J 2005;26:298-307.
3. Moons P, Van Deyk K, De Geest S, Gewillig M, Budts W. Is the severity of congenital heart disease associated with the quality of life and perceived health of adult patients? Heart 2005;91:1193- 8.
4. Moons P. Quality of life in adults with congenital heart disease: beyond the quantity of life. Leuven' Author; 2004.
5. Fekkes M, Kamphuis RP, Ottenkamp J, Verrips E, Vogels T, Kamphuis M, et al. Health-related quality of life in young adults with minor congenital heart disease. Psychol Health 2001; 16:239-50.
6. Gersony WM, Hayes CJ, Driscoll DJ, Keane JF, Kidd L, O'Fallon WM, et al. Second natural history study of congenital heart defects. Quality of life of patients with aortic stenosis, pulmonary stenosis, or ventricular septal defect. Circulation 1993;87:152-65.
7. Meijboom F, Hess J, Szatmari A, Utens EM, McGhie J, Deckers JW, et al. Long-term follow-up (9 to 20 years) after surgical closure of atrial septal defect at a young age. Am J Cardiol 1993;72:1431- 4.
8. Meijboom F, Szatmari A, Utens E, Deckers JW, Roelandt JR, Bos E, et al. Long-term follow-up after surgical closure of ventricular septal defect in infancy and childhood. J Am Coll Cardiol 1994;24:1358- 64.
9. Meijboom F, Szatmari A, Deckers JW, Utens EM, Roelandt JR, Bos E, et al. Cardiac status and health-related quality of life in the long term after surgical repair of tetralogy of Fallot in infancy and childhood. J Thorac Cardiovasc Surg 1995;110:883- 91.
10. Meijboom F, Szatmari A, Deckers JW, Utens EM, Roelandt JR, Bos E, et al. Long-term follow-up (10 to 17 years) after Mustard repair for transposition of the great arteries. J Thorac Cardiovasc Surg 1996; 111:1158-68.
11. Saliba Z, Butera G, Bonnet D, Bonhoeffer P, Villain E, Kachaner J, et al. Quality of life and perceived health status in surviving adults with univentricular heart. Heart 2001;86:69-73.
12. Walker WT, Temple IK, Gnanapragasam JP, Goddard JR, Brown EM. Quality of life after repair of tetralogy of Fallot. Cardiol Young 2002;12:549-53.
13. Kamphuis M, Ottenkamp J, Vliegen HW, Vogels T, Zwinderman KH, Kamphuis RP, et al. Health related quality of life and health status in adult survivors with previously operated complex congenital heart disease. Heart 2002;87:356-62.
14. Lane DA, Lip GY, Millane TA. Quality of life in adults with congenital heart disease. Heart 2002;88:71-5.
15. Simko LC, McGinnis KA. Quality of life experienced by adults with congenital heart disease. AACN Clin Issues 2003;14:42-53.
16. Moons P, De Geest S, Budts W. Comprehensive care for adults with congenital heart disease: expanding roles for nurses. Eur J Cardiovasc Nurs 2002;1:23- 8.
17. Simko LC. Adults with congenital heart disease: utilizing quality of life and Husted's nursing theory as a conceptual framework. Crit Care Nurs Q 1999;22:1-11.
18. Meeberg GA. Quality of life: a concept analysis. J Adv Nurs 1993; 18:32- 8.
19. Zhan L. Quality of life: conceptual and measurement issues. J Adv Nurs 1992;17:795-800.
20. Felce D. Defining and applying the concept of quality of life. J Intellect Disabil Res 1997;41(Pt 2):126-35.
21. Ferrans CE. Quality of life: conceptual issues. Semin Oncol Nurs 1990;6:248-54.
22. Haas BK. A multidisciplinary concept analysis of quality of life. West J Nurs Res 1999;21:728- 42.
23. Haas BK. Clarification and integration of similar quality of life concepts. Image J Nurs Sch 1999;31:215- 20.
24. Stewart A. Conceptual and methodologic issues in defining quality of life: state of the art. Prog Cardiovasc Nurs 1992;7:3-11.

25. Kleinpell RM. Concept analysis of quality of life. Dimens Crit Care Nurs 1991;10:223–9.
26. Antonovsky A. Unraveling the mystery of health: how people manage stress and stay well. San Fransisco' Jossey-Bass; 1987.
27. Mowad L. Correlates of quality of life in older adult veterans. West J Nurs Res 2004;26:293–306.
28. Gibson LM, Parker V. Inner resources as predictors of psychological well-being in middle-income African American breast cancer survivors. Cancer Control 2003;10:52–9.
29. Nasermoaddeli A, Sekine M, Hamanishi S, Kagamimori S. Associations between sense of coherence and psychological work characteristics with changes in quality of life in Japanese civil servants: a 1-year follow-up study. Ind Health 2003;41:236–41.
30. O'Carroll RE, Ayling R, O'Reilly SM, North NT. Alexithymia and sense of coherence in patients with total spinal cord transection. Psychosom Med 2003;65:151–5.
31. Dantas RA, Motzer SA, Ciol MA. The relationship between quality of life, sense of coherence and self-esteem in persons after coronary artery bypass graft surgery. Int J Nurs Stud 2002;39:745–55.
32. Jakobsson L. Indwelling catheter treatment and health-related quality of life in men with prostate cancer in comparison with men with benign prostatic hyperplasia. Scand J Caring Sci 2002;16:264–71.
33. Vinson JA. Children with asthma: initial development of the child resilience model. Pediatr Nurs 2002;28:149–58.
34. Ekman I, Fagerberg B, Lundman B. Health-related quality of life and sense of coherence among elderly patients with severe chronic heart failure in comparison with healthy controls. Heart Lung 2002;31: 94–101.
35. Soderman AC, Bergenius J, Bagger-Sjoback D, Tjell C, Langius A. Patients' subjective evaluations of quality of life related to diseasespecific symptoms, sense of coherence, and treatment in Meniere's disease. Otol Neurotol 2001;22:526–33.
36. Bengtsson-Tops A, Hansson L. The validity of Antonovsky's sense of coherence measure in a sample of schizophrenic patients living in the community. J Adv Nurs 2001;33:432–8.
37. Cederfjall C, Langius-Eklof A, Lidman K, Wredling R. Gender differences in perceived health-related quality of life among patients with HIV infection. AIDS Patient Care STDS 2001;15:31–9.
38. Klevsgard R, Risberg BO, Thomsen MB, Hallberg IR. A 1-year follow-up quality of life study after hemodynamically successful or unsuccessful surgical revascularization of lower limb ischemia. J Vasc Surg 2001;33:114–22.
39. Klevsgard R, Hallberg IR, Risberg B, Thomsen MB. The effects of successful intervention on quality of life in patients with varying degrees of lower-limb ischaemia. Eur J Vasc Endovasc Surg 2000;19: 238–45.
40. Nesbitt BJ, Heidrich SM. Sense of coherence and illness appraisal in older women's quality of life. Res Nurs Health 2000;23:25–34.
41. Schnyder U, Buchi S, Sensky T, Klaghofer R. Antonovsky's sense of coherence: trait or state? Psychother Psychosom 2000;69:296–302.
42. Lindstrom B, Eriksson M. Salutogenesis. J Epidemiol Community Health 2005;59:440–2.
43. Karlsson I, Berglin E, Larsson PA. Sense of coherence: quality of life before and after coronary artery bypass surgery—a longitudinal study. J Adv Nurs 2000;31:1383–92.
44. Forsberg A, Backman L, Svensson E. Liver transplant recipients' ability to cope during the first 12 months after transplantation—a prospective study. Scand J Caring Sci 2002;16:345–52.
45. Snekkevik H, Anke AG, Stanghelle JK, Fugl-Meyer AR. Is sense of coherence stable after multiple trauma? Clin Rehabil 2003;17: 443–53.
46. Wolff AC, Ratner PA. Stress, social support, and sense of coherence. West J Nurs Res 1999;21:182–97.
47. Sagy S, Antonovsky H. The development of the sense of coherence: a retrospective study of early life experiences in the family. Int J Aging Hum Dev 2000;51:155–66.
48. Claessens P, Moons P, de Casterle BD, Cannaerts N, Budts W, Gewillig M. What does it mean to live with a congenital heart disease? A qualitative study on the lived experiences of adult patients. Eur J Cardiovasc Nurs 2005;4:3–10.

 *Epilogue*

The studies described in this book show that persons with congenital heart disease can have an excellent quality of life. Their quality of life is often better than that of healthy individuals. This finding may be counterintuitive, but the study results demonstrated that these persons' quality of life is mainly determined by other factors than their heart condition. Furthermore, it is hypothesized that growing up with congenital heart disease is a generalized resistance resource which may contribute to the development of a strong sense of coherence, which in turn is associated with a good quality of life.

To test this hypothesis, a longitudinal study in adolescents and emerging adults is set-up at the Katholieke Universiteit Leuven, Belgium. The first results show, indeed, that sense of coherence is higher in persons with congenital heart disease compared to healthy control persons. This higher sense of coherence is explaining the better quality of life in persons with congenital heart disease.

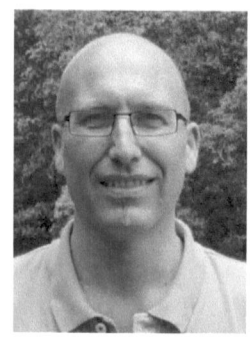

Dr. Philip Moons is Professor in Nursing Science at the Center for Health Services and Nursing Research at the Catholic University Leuven (Belgium); Advanced Practice Nurse in Congenital Cardiology at the University Hospitals Leuven (Belgium); and guest professor at the Heart Centre of Copenhagen University Hospital (Denmark).

He received his Master's Degree in nursing science from the Catholic University Leuven in 1995, and obtained his PhD in 2004 from the same university. Philip Moons is mainly involved in outcome and quality of life research in congenital heart disease, and developed and implemented the role of advanced practice nurse in the Adult Congenital Heart Disease Program of the University Hospital of Leuven.

For his work, Philip Moons received Martha N. Hill New Investigators Award 2004 from the American Heart Association and the Atie Immink New Investigators Award 2008 from the European Society of Cardiology. He is fellow of the American Heart Association (FAHA), the European Society of Cardiology (NFESC), and the European Academy of Nursing Science (FEANS). Philip Moons has published more than 130 articles in international, peer-reviewed journals; and presented more than 180 abstracts at national and international conferences.

perswww.kuleuven.be/~u0032865

www.ingramcontent.com/pod-product-compliance
Ingram Content Group UK Ltd.
Pitfield, Milton Keynes, MK11 3LW, UK
UKHW041958230426
12048UKWH00008B/410